Adolescent Cannabis Use

Editors

PAULA RIGGS
JESSE D. HINCKLEY
J. MEGAN ROSS

PSYCHIATRIC CLINICS OF NORTH AMERICA

www.psych.theclinics.com

Consulting Editor
HARSH K. TRIVEDI

December 2023 • Volume 46 • Number 4

ELSEVIER

1600 John F. Kennedy Boulevard • Suite 1800 • Philadelphia, Pennsylvania, 19103-2899

http://www.theclinics.com

PSYCHIATRIC CLINICS OF NORTH AMERICA Volume 46, Number 4
December 2023 ISSN 0193-953X, ISBN-13: 978-0-443-12893-6

Editor: Megan Ashdown
Developmental Editor: Malvika Shah

Psychiatric Clinics of North America (ISSN 0193-953X) is published quarterly by Elsevier Inc., 360 Park Avenue South, New York, NY 10010-1710. Months of issue are March, June, September, and December. Business and Editorial Offices: 1600 John F. Kennedy Blvd., Suite 1800, Philadelphia, PA 19103-2899. Periodicals postage paid at New York, NY and additional mailing offices. Subscription prices are $352.00 per year (US individuals), $781.00 per year (US institutions), $100.00 per year (US students/residents), $422.00 per year (Canadian individuals), $519.00 per year (international individuals), $983.00 per year (Canadian & international institutions), and $220.00 per year (international students/residents), $100.00 per year (Canadian & students/residents). Foreign air speed delivery is included in all *Clinics'* subscription prices. All prices are subject to change without notice. **POSTMASTER:** Send address changes to *Psychiatric Clinics of North America*, Elsevier Health Sciences Division, Subscription Customer Service, 3251 Riverport Lane, Maryland Heights, MO 63043. **Customer Service: 1-800-654-2452 (US). From outside the United States, call 1-314-447-8871. Fax: 1-314-447-8029. E-mail: journalscustomerservice-usa@elsevier.com (for print support)** and **journalsonlinesupport-usa@elsevier.com (for online support).**

Reprints. For copies of 100 or more, of articles in this publication, please contact the Commercial Reprints Department, Elsevier Inc., 360 Park Avenue South, New York, New York 10010-1710. Tel.: 212-633-3874, Fax: 212-633-3820, E-mail: reprints@elsevier.com.

Psychiatric Clinics of North America is covered in *MEDLINE/PubMed (Index Medicus), Current Contents/Social and Behavioral Sciences, Social Science Citation Index, Embase/Excerpta Medica,* and PsycINFO.

Contributors

CONSULTING EDITOR

HARSH K. TRIVEDI, MD, MBA
President and Chief Executive Officer, Sheppard Pratt, Clinical Professor of Psychiatry, University of Maryland School of Medicine, Baltimore, Maryland

EDITORS

PAULA RIGGS, MD
Professor, Director, Division of Addiction Science, Prevention, and Treatment, Department of Psychiatry, University of Colorado School of Medicine, Aurora, Colorado

JESSE D. HINCKLEY, MD, PhD
Assistant Professor, Director of Adolescent Psychiatric Services, ARTS, Co-Director of the Addiction Biology Lab, Division of Addiction Science, Prevention, and Treatment, Department of Psychiatry, University of Colorado School of Medicine, Aurora, Colorado

J. MEGAN ROSS, PhD
Assistant Professor, Division of Addiction Science, Prevention, and Treatment, Department of Psychiatry, University of Colorado School of Medicine, Aurora, Colorado

AUTHORS

ZACHARY W. ADAMS, PhD
Assistant Professor, Department of Psychiatry, Indiana University School of Medicine, Indianapolis, Indiana

DEVIKA BHATIA, MD
Instructor, University of Colorado, Aurora, Colorado

QUANDRA BLACKENEY, BS
Center for the Clinical Trials Network, National Institute on Drug Abuse, Bethesda, Maryland

JESSICA B. CALIHAN, MD, MS
Division of Adolescent and Young Adult Medicine, Boston Children's Hospital, Boston, Massachusetts

MICHELLE CORBIN, MBA
Center for the Clinical Trials Network, National Institute on Drug Abuse, Bethesda, Maryland

KENYATTA CRENSHAW, MEd
The Bizzell Group LLC, New Carrollton, Maryland

KEVIN GRAY, MD
Professor of Psychiatry and Behavioral Sciences and Assistant Provost for Research Advancement, Medical University of South Carolina, Charleston, South Carolina

DANIEL HASHEMI, MD
Resident Physician, Department of Psychiatry and Behavioral Sciences, Medical University of South Carolina, Charleston, South Carolina

JESSE D. HINCKLEY, MD, PhD
Assistant Professor, Division of Addiction Science, Treatment, and Prevention, Department of Psychiatry, University of Colorado School of Medicine, Aurora, Colorado

HYMAN HOPS, PhD
Senior Scientist, Oregon Research Institute, Eugene, Oregon; Albuquerque, New Mexico

LESLIE A. HULVERSHORN, MD
Associate Professor, Department of Psychiatry, Indiana University School of Medicine, Indianapolis, Indiana

KRISTEN HUNTLEY, PhD
Center for the Clinical Trials Network, National Institute on Drug Abuse, Bethesda, Maryland

KRISTIE LADEGARD, MD
Assistant Professor, Denver Health, University of Colorado, Denver, Colorado

SHARON LEVY, MD, MPH
Associate Professor of Pediatrics, Harvard Medical School, Division of Addiction Medicine, Boston Children's Hospital, Harvard Medical School, Boston, Massachusetts

JANET LINTON, MSM
Center for the Clinical Trials Network, National Institute on Drug Abuse, Bethesda, Maryland

TODD MANDELL, MD
The Bizzell Group LLC, New Carrollton, Maryland

BRIGID R. MARRIOTT, PhD
Postdoctoral Fellow, Department of Psychiatry, Indiana University School of Medicine, Indianapolis, Indiana

KARLA MOLINERO, MD
Addiction Psychiatry Fellow, Department of Psychiatry, University of Colorado School of Medicine, Aurora, Colorado

ALEAH MONTANO, BA
Project Coordinator, Oregon Research Institute, Eugene, Oregon; Albuquerque, New Mexico

KAYLA M. NELSON, BS
Institute of Child Development, University of Minnesota, Minneapolis, Minnesota

LAURA NOLAN, BA
JBS International, Inc, North Bethesda, Maryland

TIM OZECHOWSKI, PhD
Senior Scientist, Oregon Research Institute, Eugene, Oregon

PAULA RIGGS, MD
Professor and Vice-Chair, Faculty Affairs, Director, Division of Addiction Sciences, Prevention, and Treatment, Department of Psychiatry, University of Colorado School of Medicine, University of Colorado Anschutz Medical Campus, Aurora, Colorado

J. MEGAN ROSS, PhD
Assistant Professor, Department of Psychiatry, Division of Addiction Sciences, University of Colorado Anschutz Medical Campus, Aurora, Colorado

JONATHAN D. SCHAEFER, PhD
Institute of Child Development, University of Minnesota, Minneapolis, Minnesota

J. COBB SCOTT, PhD
Department of Psychiatry, Perelman School of Medicine, University of Pennsylvania, VISN4 Mental Illness Research, Education, and Clinical Center at the Corporal Michael J. Crescenz VA Medical Center, Philadelphia, Pennsylvania

SHADI SHARIF, BA
Department of Psychiatry, University of Colorado School of Medicine, Aurora, Colorado

GEETHA A. SUBRAMANIAM, MD
Center for the Clinical Trials Network, National Institute on Drug Abuse, Bethesda, Maryland

ABIGAIL L. TUVEL, BA
Institute for Behavioral Genetics, University of Colorado Boulder, Boulder, Colorado

HOLLY WALDRON, PhD
Senior Scientist, Oregon Research Institute, Eugene, Oregon; Albuquerque, New Mexico

MICHELLE L. WEST, PhD
Assistant Professor, Department of Psychiatry, University of Colorado School of Medicine, Aurora, Colorado

SYLIA WILSON, PhD
Institute of Child Development, University of Minnesota, Minneapolis, Minnesota

EVAN A. WINIGER, PhD
Department of Psychiatry, University of Colorado Anschutz Medical Campus, Aurora, Colorado

KEN C. WINTERS, PhD
Senior Scientist, Oregon Research Institute, Eugene, Oregon

Contents

Because of substantial limitations in available national data, such as inconsistencies among surveys and small sample sizes, the increased prevalence of cannabis use among adolescents since recreational legalization has not been directly observed. Nevertheless, both usage frequency and product potency have significantly increased, alongside alternative routes of delivery to smoking, such as vaping cannabis. Moreover, certain populations may be especially vulnerable to the effects of legalization. Regardless of differing state-level cannabis legalization status, the adverse consequences of cannabis on youth have clear negative impacts on mental health, medical symptoms, educational outcomes, and increased risk of addiction to other substances.

With increasing cannabis potency, increasing variety of methods of cannabis use, and lower perceived risk of cannabis use, it is increasingly important clinicians who work with adolescents remain up-to-date on the latest literature regarding cannabis use and its associated outcomes. Adolescent cannabis use is associated with chronic cognitive, psychosocial, psychiatric, and physical outcomes. Clinicians working in this field should be able to recognize cannabis use disorder, understand how adolescent cannabis use can impact the developing mind, and have informed discussions with patients and families regarding risks of use.

Research examining associations between frequent cannabis use in adolescence and brain-behavior outcomes has increased substantially over the past 2 decades. This review attempts to synthesize the state of evidence in this area of research while acknowledging challenges in interpretation. Although there is converging evidence that ongoing, frequent cannabis use in adolescence is associated with small reductions in cognitive functioning, there is still significant debate regarding the persistence of reductions after a period of abstinence. Similarly, there is controversy regarding the replicability of structural and functional neuroimaging findings related to frequent cannabis use in adolescence. Larger studies with informative designs are needed.

Research has led to the development of hundreds of evidence-based prevention interventions, most of which are school-based prevention programs. Most primary care clinicians and child/adolescent behavioral health clinicians are unfamiliar with and/or lack training in evidence-based prevention interventions. However, most clinicians in these settings routinely screen children for developmental delays and skills deficits that increase the risk of developing substance abuse and a broad range of mental health and behavior problems by adolescence. It is hoped that the broader use of these practical evidence-based prevention tools may expand the prevention workforce to address the current youth mental health crisis.

Adolescent cannabis use is a modifiable health behavior with potential adverse developmental, cognitive, psychological, and health effects. Over the last 2 decades, work to promote implementation of screening, brief intervention, and referral to treatment has improved screening, use of validated screening tools, and preventive messaging. Current intervention strategies for cannabis use are associated with modest, short-term effects, and referral to treatment is limited by availability of resources for adolescent substance use. This article provides an update on the evidence base for screening, brief intervention, referral to treatment, and the current state of implementation focused on management of cannabis use disorder.

This article discusses the application of brief interventions to address adolescents with a cannabis use problem. Topics include a general model of brief interventions, the outcome literature, existing brief interventions that focus on youth cannabis use, adjustments to a brief intervention when addressing cannabis, referral to treatment issues, personalizing a brief intervention, the need to address coexisting problems, and future directions.

This review summarizes treatments for cannabis use disorder (CUD) in adolescents. The best supported CUD treatments are cognitive behavioral psychotherapies, including family-based models that facilitate environmental changes and youth-focused models that incorporate skills training, motivational interviewing, and contingency management to promote reductions in cannabis use. Some medications show promise in reducing cannabis craving and withdrawal symptoms. Further research is needed on the efficacy and implementation of existing treatments given the changes in cannabis use trends over time and on emerging technologies that may expand access to evidence-based CUD treatments.

Geetha A. Subramaniam, Laura Nolan, Kristen Huntley, Michelle Corbin, Kenyatta Crenshaw, Todd Mandell, Janet Linton, and Quandra Blackeney

The wide and effective dissemination of research findings is crucial to the mission of the National Institute on Drug Abuse (NIDA). This article describes NIDA dissemination efforts and resources that are available to inform clinicians, teens, families, and educators about youth and substance use. Resources that are available include content addressing facts about youth drug use, trends in use, and stigma, in addition to substance use disorder (SUD) prevention and treatment. Information is provided about resources such as infographics, research-based practice guides, training, educational events, and online videos. How input is solicited to inform dissemination efforts is described and future directions for NIDA's dissemination efforts are outlined.

Paula Riggs

PSYCHIATRIC CLINICS OF NORTH AMERICA

SERIES OF RELATED INTEREST

Child and Adolescent Psychiatric Clinics of North America
https://www.childpsych.theclinics.com/

Neurologic Clinics
https://www.neurologic.theclinics.com/

Advances in Psychiatry and Behavioral Health
https://www.advancesinpsychiatryandbehavioralhealth.com/

THE CLINICS ARE AVAILABLE ONLINE!
Access your subscription at:
www.theclinics.com

Preface

Addressing Cannabis Use During Adolescence

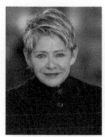
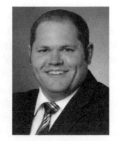
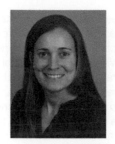

Paula Riggs, MD	Jesse D. Hinckley, MD, PhD	J. Megan Ross, PhD
	Editors	

Cannabis is among the most common substances used by adolescents. While other substance use, including alcohol and cigarette use, has declined over the past two decades, the prevalence of cannabis use has remained steady among adolescents and increased among young adults. Furthermore, over the past decade, there has been a dramatic rise in the prevalence of vaping, including nicotine and cannabis. While the prevalence of cannabis use appears to have remained steady among adolescents, Δ9-tetrahydrocannabinol (THC) potency has risen sharply, with compensatory changes in the THC/cannabidiol ratio.

Adolescence is a period of unique vulnerability to the adverse neurodevelopmental consequences of cannabis use, with potential long-term cognitive and mental health concerns. Yet, many clinicians do not feel confident discussing the impact of cannabis use with adolescents, and the majority of adolescents with cannabis use disorder (CUD) are not referred for treatment.

Mental health professionals have a vital role to play in educating adolescents, families, and clinicians, as well as other allied professionals and policy-makers, about the consequences of adolescent cannabis use. Furthermore, mental health clinics are well-situated to integrate best practices for screening and CUD treatment, as cannabis use often cooccurs with and complicates other mental health disorders. Addressing cannabis use in child and adolescent mental health settings is particularly important, as the individuals most vulnerable to the negative consequences of cannabis use appear to be adolescents with underlying mental health disorders, minority

This article originally appeared in Child and Adolescent Psychiatric Clinics, Volume 32 Issue 1, January 2023.

Psychiatr Clin N Am 46 (2023) xiii–xv
https://doi.org/10.1016/j.psc.2023.06.018
0193-953X/23/© 2023 Published by Elsevier Inc.

adolescents, adolescents who identify as LGBTQ+, and young women who are pregnant or nursing. Especially over the past decade, the body of literature exploring the impacts of recreational cannabis legalization, the impacts of cannabis on adolescent development, mental health, and other outcomes; and evidence-based screening, brief intervention, and treatment practices has expanded. While much of what is known is observational, and causal inferences cannot be made, this growing body of literature highlights key clinical findings and proposes evidence-based interventions and treatments.

This issue presents the current state of cannabis research among adolescents to meaningfully present up-to-date information for clinicians. In their article, Ladegard and Bhatia describe the impact of recreational cannabis legalization on adolescent cannabis use. While there are notable limitations to studies of cannabis legalization, there are several key findings that should be considered throughout this issue. While prevalence of cannabis use appears to have remained steady among adolescents aged 12 to 17 years, it has increased among young adults aged 18 to 25 years. Furthermore, the impact of cannabis legalization on the frequency of cannabis use and the amount of cannabis consumed remains unknown. The authors also review other potential impacts of cannabis legalization, including decreased perceived harmfulness, increased prevalence of CUD among adolescents, and increased THC potency and availability of high-potency products.

We next present a series of articles that discuss specific outcomes of adolescent cannabis use. Hashemi and Gray provide a clinical review of CUD in adolescents in which the authors review key clinical aspects of the endocannabinoid system and the impact of cannabis use, the acute and chronic physiologic effects of cannabis use, cannabis withdrawal, and the clinical features and diagnosis of CUD and severity. In this context, the authors also consider the impact of cannabis policy changes and consequent cannabis product and adolescent perception changes on CUD. Next, Scott explores the impact of adolescent cannabis use on neurocognitive and brain development, including the residual effects of cannabis use on cognitive functioning, brain structure, and brain function. As Scott discusses, while many findings need replication and further study, there remain concerns that adolescent-onset, sustained cannabis use may result in cognitive deficits and that some deficits may not recover with abstinence. In an article on psychosocial functioning, Shaefer, Nelson, and Wilson evaluate the impact of cannabis use on peer and romantic relationships, parent-child relationships, school performance and educational attainment, adult socioeconomic status, and legal consequences. As the authors highlight, most studies are observational, a common limitation in adolescent cannabis research, and the mechanisms by which cannabis use affects cannabis use remain unknown.

Next, Molinero and Hinckley review comorbid CUD and attention-deficit/hyperactivity disorder (ADHD), and West and Sharif review cooccurring cannabis use and psychosis, two challenging clinical topics in adolescent cannabis use. In the former, Molinero and Hinckley outline the overlap between cannabis use, ADHD, and other internalizing and externalizing disorders and propose evidence-based guidelines for treating these comorbid conditions. Next, West and Sharif explore the overlap of cannabis use and psychosis, outlining an approach to assessment and treatment. This section concludes with an article by Tuvel, Winnegar, and Ross reviewing the effects of adolescent cannabis use on physical health. Implicated systems include the pulmonary, cardiovascular, gastrointestinal, and endocrine systems, as well as notable impacts on complex traits, such as body mass index and sleep.

The penultimate section reviews evidence-based strategies to prevent and address problematic cannabis use and treat CUD in adolescents. Riggs presents an innovative approach to prevention, focusing on antecedent risk factors and skills deficits and identifying evidence-based prevention tools. Next, Calihan and Levy outline the principles of screening, brief intervention, and referral to treatment, the current standard of care for all adolescents in primary care and mental health settings. Herein, the authors provide important clinical resources and explore implementation in specific clinical settings. Winters, Waldron, Hopps, Ozechowski, and Montano then expand on brief interventions for adolescents with problematic cannabis use. The authors outline the application of brief intervention, supported by review of the literature, to address individual adolescent needs and facilitate referral to treatment as indicated. In the following article, Adams, Marriott, Hulvershorn, and Hinckley review evidence-based treatment of CUD in adolescents. Notably, the primary interventions are therapy-based, with N-acetyl cysteine being effective in promoting abstinence during treatment.

This issue concludes with an article by Subramaniam, Nolan, Huntley, Corbin, Crenshaw, Mandell, Linton, and Blackeney outlining efforts by the National Institute on Drug Abuse (NIDA) to disseminate scientific knowledge and clinical resources to address adolescent cannabis use. NIDA has developed resources specifically for clinicians, adolescents, parents, and trusted adults that are readily available in cost-free print and digital formats.

We hope this issue provides a valuable resource on the state of cannabis use research in adolescents to empower clinicians to discuss the impacts of cannabis use on adolescents and to engage adolescents in evidence-based interventions. Adolescent cannabis research is a rapidly evolving field, with policy changes outpacing research over the past decade. It is imperative for clinicians to remain up-to-date and proactively engage adolescents and families.

Paula Riggs, MD
Division of Addiction Science, Prevention and Treatment, Department of Psychiatry, University of Colorado School of Medicine, 1890 North Revere Court, MS-F570, Aurora, CO 80045, USA

Jesse D. Hinckley, MD, PhD
Division of Addiction Science, Prevention and Treatment, Department of Psychiatry, University of Colorado School of Medicine, 1890 North Revere Court, MS-F570, Aurora, CO 80045, USA

J. Megan Ross, PhD
Division of Addiction Science, Prevention and Treatment, Department of Psychiatry, University of Colorado School of Medicine, 1890 North Revere Court, MS-F570, Aurora, CO 80045, USA

E-mail addresses:
PAULA.RIGGS@CUANSCHUTZ.EDU (P. Riggs)
JESSE.HINCKLEY@CUANSCHUTZ.EDU (J.D. Hinckley)
JESSICA.M.ROSS@CUANSCHUTZ.EDU (J.M. Ross)

Impact of Cannabis Legalization on Adolescent Cannabis Use

Kristie Ladegard, MD[a],*, Devika Bhatia, MD[b]

KEYWORDS

- Cannabis legalization • Adolescent • Cannabis • Policy • Substance use • Minority

KEY POINTS

- Most research on medical legalization and youth cannabis use has found no substantial changes in usage, although patterns of use may have increased. Nevertheless, these population surveys do not capture the nuances of varied state regulations and their effects.
- Recreational legalization has been linked to increased variation in different cannabis usage mediums. These include the increase of cannabis products with significantly higher psychoactive potency, such as vaping.
- Future studies should aim to explore nuances in differences of implementation of recreational and medical legalization laws and their effects on adolescent cannabis use as well as other unintended consequences of cannabis legalization.

INTRODUCTION

Cannabis use among adolescents is increasing. In recent years, several studies have observed past-month usage at more than 20% among youth, including an age-period-cohort analysis that observed the strongest age effects in this group.[1] This contrasts with an overall downward trend in adolescent substance use during the last 2 decades.[2] Importantly, as of January 2022, 36 states have legalized medical cannabis, and 18 of those have legalized recreational cannabis. Although sales of recreational cannabis have been age-limited, and legalization laws differ by state (eg, medical cannabis vs recreational cannabis, merchant availability, legal enforcement), the consequences of legalization on adolescent cannabis use remain an area of concern. Developmentally, adolescence is a period of time during which many substance use disorders emerge.[3] The cannabinoid system plays an important role in brain development, particularly during adolescence when the brain is still developing and sensitive to environmental disturbances.[1]

This article originally appeared in *Child and Adolescent Psychiatric Clinics*, Volume 32 Issue 1, January 2023.
[a] Denver Health, University of Colorado, 601 Broadway 7th Floor, MC7779, Denver, CO 80203, USA; [b] University of Colorado, 13007 East 19th Place, Aurora, CO 80045, USA
* Corresponding author.
E-mail address: kristie.ladegard@dhha.org

Understanding how legalization affects adolescent cannabis usage poises clinicians and policymakers to create more effective, targeted interventions. This review thus aims to comprehensively describe and discuss the impacts of cannabis legalization on adolescent cannabis use (both in prevalence and in altered patterns) and other unintended consequences for this vulnerable population. Specifically, the authors discuss trends in adolescent cannabis use, perceptions of cannabis, routes and modes of use, health and safety concerns, and impacts on special populations following medical legalization and recreational legalization.

OVERALL TRENDS IN ADOLESCENT CANNABIS USE
Medical Legalization

As state-level medical legalization preceded recreational legalization of cannabis, more information is available on the effects that medical legalization has had on adolescent cannabis use. Most studies assessing medical legalization and adolescent cannabis use (lifetime or past-month cannabis use) have found no significant changes in adolescent cannabis use,[4–6] although patterns of use may have been affected.[7,8] For instance, nationally representative data from the Monitoring the Future study indicated that adolescent cannabis use decreased among 8th graders (0.2%–2.4% decrease) and was not statistically significant different among 10th and 12th graders following medical legalization.[4]

Several studies have examined variations in adolescent cannabis usage, such as incidence of cannabis use disorder (CUD), frequency/potency of cannabis use, and cannabis use initiation. A prior study also investigated whether there were significant increases in cannabis usage frequency, an indication of possible CUD; states with medicinal marijuana laws had a greater percentage of people who used cannabis in the last 30 days (5.44%) compared with nonlegal states (4.15%).[7] A nationally representative sample demonstrated that youth aged 12 to 20 years old were more likely to experiment with cannabis if living in a state in which medical cannabis was legal.[8] Moreover, in a study with 80 adolescents in outpatient substance abuse treatment in Colorado, up to 48.8% of participants reported acquiring cannabis from someone with a medical cannabis license.[9] Understanding the nuances specific for cannabis-related behaviors and outcomes as a result of medical legalization is vital for identifying risks for the adolescent population.

Recreational Legalization

Recreational cannabis legalization is a relatively new phenomenon. Initially, a few studies evaluated state-level data of early adopters of recreational legalization and its effects on adolescent cannabis use. For instance, 1 study investigated high school students' cannabis use patterns before/after initiation of retail sales of cannabis in Colorado (January 2014) and found a significant decrease in perceived harmfulness following recreational enactment (52.9%–47.7%; $P<.01$), although no significant changes in perceived accessibility, wrongfulness, or parental disapproval.[2] Small but significant increases in usage were observed in Washington 8th and 10th graders (2% and 4% increases, respectively) as well.[10]

As more states legalize recreational cannabis, more data will be available for further examination of nationally representative data sets. A 2020 study described modest but significant increases in CUD among adolescents aged 12 to 17 years old (2.18% to 2.72%), with larger increases in CUD among past-year cannabis users (22.8%–27.2%) following recreational cannabis legalization.[11] By contrast, a study conducted in 2021 used Youth Risk Behavior Surveillance data, providing no statistically significant change in past-30-day use or frequent use (used at least 10 times during past 30 days) following recreational legalization law enactment.[12] In addition, it is important to consider the young adult population, for whom purchase of recreational cannabis is legal; per National Survey on Drug Use and Health data, 18- to 25-year-olds in cannabis-legal states experienced a 48% increase in past-30-day cannabis use compared with young adults in nonlegal states, who experienced an 18% increase in use in the same time period.[13] The longer-term impacts of recreational legalization on adolescent cannabis usage patterns will need to be continuously assessed, as distinctions in legal cannabis policies persist between state-level jurisdictions.

Perceptions of Cannabis

Tracking societal perceptions of cannabis use before and after legalization is imperative owing to the impact it may have on teens' views of cannabis. Several recent studies have shown declines in perceived harmfulness of cannabis use corresponding to implementation of legal recreational cannabis.[10,14-18] Adolescent perceptions of cannabis as a harmful substance are at an all-time low, regardless of state.[19,20] Furthermore, youth attitudes toward cannabis have been trending toward greater acceptance of use, and the perceived risk of regularly smoking cannabis has significantly declined, according to the Monitoring Future Survey.[21]

It is also vital to examine into how legalization changes parents' attitudes toward cannabis, given their major influence on their children's health behaviors. Use of adolescent cannabis has been linked to greater parental use and favorable parental perceptions postlegalization.[22,23] Moreover, a study in Colorado indicated that parents frequently talked to their children about cannabis but did not discuss its risks and health effects.[24] In legal states, parents may struggle to communicate the risks of cannabis usage to their children owing to conflicting messages from media and society about its benefits. In the same Colorado survey, only 30% of adolescents said a doctor had discussed cannabis use with them.[24] These findings highlight the need for public education programs to accompany cannabis legalization, in order to raise awareness of the negative consequences of cannabis use.

Routes, Modes of Use, and Potency Levels

Smoking cannabis is the most common mode of use among youths. According to national cross-sectional data, almost 80% of adolescent cannabis users reported smoking it within the past month.[25] Nonetheless, cannabis legalization has been associated with increased potency of cannabis products and the rise of increasingly potent products alongside the diversification of ways of consumption (eg, vaporizing devices, edibles).[26,27] Over the last decade, the National Institute on Drug Abuse has evaluated more than 18,000 samples of cannabis products as part of a potency monitoring program.[28] The findings indicated that the mean concentration of 9-tetrahydrocannabinol (THC) has increased significantly in recent years from 8.9% in 2008 to 17.1% in 2017.

Although plant matter of cannabis contains variable concentrations of THC, recent data suggest that adolescents who vape cannabis most often use highly potent cannabis oil, wax, or liquid preparations.[29] Furthermore, in cannabis-legal states, adolescents have higher rates of using edibles (51.4% vs 37.2% in nonlegal states) and concentrates (22.0% vs 15.4% in nonlegal states), although dried herb continues to be more prevalent in nonlegal states (80.8% in nonlegal states vs 77.7% in legal states).[6] The increase of using significantly higher potency butane hash oil or "dab" or "shatter" has also raised concern for adverse effects on adolescents,[30] especially as its use has been associated with acute psychosis and cardiotoxicity.[31,32]

A study examining the association between cannabis legalization and adolescent cannabis use methods found that legalization for a longer period of time and higher dispensary density were associated with higher rates of adolescents trying edibles or electronic vapor product use.[33] Furthermore, data from the Youth Risk Tobacco Survey indicate that adolescents in cannabis-legal states are more likely to use cannabis in electronic vapor products compared with adolescents in states in which cannabis is not legal.[34] Studies additionally suggest that parental use of cannabis with children in the home has increased from 4.9% to 6.8% from 2002 to 2015,[35] which has implications for increased risk for accidental ingestion by children in the home as well as second-hand smoke exposure. Clinicians in recreational-legal states should discuss these adverse outcomes with patients and parents.

IMPLICATIONS FOR ADOLESCENT HEALTH AND DEVELOPMENT
Cognitive Development

In states with recreational cannabis laws, younger adolescents (13–16 years old compared with 17 years old) had an elevated adjusted odds of cannabis-related hospitalizations across the study years, which may indicate earlier cannabis commencement among adolescents.[36] This is particularly concerning given that neurocognitive impairment at young adulthood has been linked to a younger age of initiation and more regular cannabis usage at 14 years and throughout adolescence.[37] Indeed, several important studies in child development suggest that the adolescent brain is highly susceptible to the neurotoxic effects of cannabis, especially in terms of neurocognitive functioning. Cognitive deficits produced by cannabis have shown decreased performance on measures of spatial working memory, verbal and episodic memory, complex attention executive function (eg, decision making, planning, inhibitory, control), and processing speed.[38] In a longitudinal study of greater than 1000 children observed from infancy to adulthood, those who used cannabis frequently during adolescence had the lowest IQ scores.[39]

Academic Performance

Adolescent cannabis use frequency and onset age have been linked to lower rates of graduation from high school, even when including controls for alcohol and tobacco use, and external issues.[38] Studies suggest that impaired functioning on measures of psychomotor speed, emotional control, learning, memory, and executive function is consistent with findings of lower grades, higher absenteeism, lower scholastic aptitude test scores, greater reported school difficulty, and decreased college degree attainment observed in cannabis-using adolescents and young adults.[40] A rigorous analysis of 4 large epidemiologic trials found that cannabis use during adolescence is also associated with reductions in the odds of high school completion and degree attainment in a dose-dependent fashion, which suggests that cannabis use is causative.[41]

School suspensions and expulsions for substance use further hinder graduation and academic performance. Since recreational cannabis was legalized in 2012, the number of Colorado high school students suspended for cannabis has increased from 17% to 23%.[42] Moreover, even though suspensions in Colorado did decrease during COVID-19 in 2019 to 2020 and 2020 to 2021, cannabis was still the number one reason for law enforcement contact in Colorado for schools during this time.[43] Cannabis use is also influenced by a school's drug use disciplinary rules. Indeed, adapting remedial methods for conduct violations involving cannabis, such as psychoeducation, has been associated with reduced use.[44] For example, clinicians who engage with school-based health centers (SBHCs) can provide adolescents with confidential counseling. Screening, brief intervention, and referral to treatment has also been adopted as a routine protocol in SBHCs in Colorado to enable early detection of at-risk adolescents.[45]

Mental Health

Adolescent exposure to cannabis predicts up to a twofold increased risk of developing psychosis and schizophrenia in adulthood.[46] This finding has been replicated multiple times in large cohort studies controlling for multiple variables, including family history, psychosis preceding cannabis use, and intoxication at the time of final assessment. This finding is also dose-dependent, meaning that the more cannabis to which youth are exposed, the greater the odds are of developing psychosis as an adult.[46]

Another possible mental health risk for youth from all races and socioeconomic groups is suicide, the second leading cause of death in people between 10 and 24 years of age.[47] Previous studies have shown an association between cannabis and suicidal behavior; heavy cannabis users have a higher incidence of suicide attempts and suicide completion.[48] Potential small but significant increases in deaths by suicide in 15- to 24-year-olds were observed in Washington State following legalization of cannabis.[49] Results from a recent meta-analysis found that cannabis consumption in adolescence is associated with a modest increase in the odds of depression, suicidal ideations, and suicide attempts in young adulthood even in the absence of a premorbid condition.[50]

As with mood and psychotic outcomes, adolescent cannabis use is also associated with increased risk for developing addictive disorders in adulthood to cannabis and other drugs. Both cross-sectional and longitudinal studies have shown a significant relationship between early-onset cannabis exposure and a greater likelihood of developing an addictive disorder.[51–54] A large longitudinal study showed that daily users of cannabis who started using before age 17 years were more likely to develop cannabis dependence and use illicit drugs.[41] The above implications concerning adolescent cannabis use and its risk for developmental and mental health challenges underscore the need for more research on the effects of legalization on adverse psychosocial outcomes.

Driving

In addition to several negative health impacts, adolescent cannabis use has also been linked to problems with driving safety. Several meta-analyses have found that cannabis significantly increases the likelihood of driving accidents. Driving performance requires divided attention, and studies with young adults have observed significantly worsened ability to drive in complex situations following cannabis use.[55] In another study investigating adolescent drivers, nearly half (48.8%) of participants reported driving after using marijuana (DAUM), and the prevalence of DAUM (12.7%) was more than twice as high compared with driving after drinking (5.0%).[56] This may reflect a perception that DAUM is less risky and more feasible compared with drunk driving. Individuals should be advised to refrain from driving for at least a 3 hours after smoking cannabis, and even longer for more potent and/or long-lasting ingestion methods. Teenagers and parents should be advised not to drive 3 hours after smoking cannabis (and even longer if using edibles). Because cannabis is frequently identified in vehicle accidents (both fatal and nonfatal), it is vital to monitor how changing laws may affect adolescent usage and driving.

Acute Care

Because adolescents with mental health and substance use challenges are routinely treated in clinical settings, the impact of cannabis legalization on cannabis-related visits to acute care clinics warrants attention. After recreational cannabis regulations were implemented in Colorado, a study observed a significant increase in adolescent cannabis-related emergency department and urgent care admissions.[57] Similarly, adolescent exposures to cannabis reported to the Rocky Mountain Poison Center increased 13.0% from 2010 to 2014, with larger increases in the number of exposures following sales of recreational cannabis in retail (76.9% increase in exposures from 2014 to 2019).[58] Increased emergency department visits and hospitalizations of adolescents have occurred in part because of higher-potency cannabis use, leading to psychosis, depression, and anxiety.[59–63] Furthermore, a large metropolitan area in California noted admissions for cyclic vomiting associated with cannabis use among teens and young adults increased following legalization of recreational cannabis.[64] The cannabis hyperemesis syndrome incidence has increased with increases in cannabis accessibility in Colorado as well.[65]

A recent retrospective cohort study of adolescent hospitalizations at children's hospitals from 2008 to 2009 identified similar trends.[36] Although cannabis-related hospitalizations in children's hospitals were increasing before policy change, postlegalization cannabis-related hospitalizations increased substantially, particularly in states with recreational cannabis laws where cannabis-related hospitalization tripled.[37] These findings suggest a fundamental link between recreational cannabis laws and adolescent cannabis-related hospitalizations.

SPECIAL POPULATIONS
Ethnic Minorities

Legalization may reduce the perceived health and social risks of cannabis use among youth, which may subsequently increase use and ultimately lead to youth being charged under the law for using cannabis. A major campaign argument advanced by proponents of cannabis legalization was that legalization would decrease arrests overall, especially for minority populations. This was not the case, however, for youth in Oregon, where the rate of juvenile cannabis allegations increased after legalization, including after adjustment for cannabis use trends among youth.[66] The largest disparity in allegations before legalization was among American Indian/Alaska Native youth relative to white youth, and this disparity remained unchanged after legalization.[67] For black youth, disparities were reduced following legalization, but allegation rates still remained greater than for white youth.[67] Results from other states suggest similar outcomes: legalization, as implemented in Alaska, Colorado, and Washington through 2016, did not reduce arrests for nonviolent possession of cannabis among youths, despite having benefited adults.[68] Juvenile arrests can have negative outcomes on youth, such as lower educational attainment and limited employment opportunities compared with their peers.[67] Thus, monitoring how legalization of cannabis may impact the legal implications for youth is imperative.

Pregnant Adolescents

Another particularly vulnerable population that may be negatively impacted by cannabis is pregnant adolescents. They may be exposed to online media sources suggesting use of cannabis to relieve nausea and vomiting during pregnancy but do not systematically present the risks and benefits. For example, 69% of dispensaries surveyed in Colorado recommended cannabis for morning sickness without listing possible risks with cannabis use during pregnancy.[69] One study found that the percentage of young women ages 12 to 22 years, enrolled in an adolescent-specific prenatal care program in Colorado from 2009 to 2015 with a positive urine toxicology screen for cannabis, was higher after legalization (16.2% vs 20.2%; OR, 1.3 (1.0–1.7); $P = .048$).[70] Cannabis use was higher following legalization, even in a population that cannot legally access it.[70] This is concerning due to the possible adverse effects cannabis can have on prenatal development of babies. A statistically significant association exists between prenatal cannabis use and low birthweight,[71] as well as a small but persistent positive association between prenatal cannabis use and neonatal intensive care unit admission.[72] Furthermore, 3 large-scale longitudinal studies that tracked how maternal cannabis use affected their child's development showed the following results: children of cannabis users were more impulsive and hyperactive and exhibited behavioral issues, lower IQ scores, and memory problems when compared with children of nonusers.[73] Therefore, clinicians should educate sexually active and pregnant teens about the adverse consequences of perinatal cannabis use.

FUTURE DIRECTIONS FOR RESEARCH

Long-term data on outcomes of early-onset cannabis use are still in the early stages, and several unknown factors remain. Future studies are needed to identify populations that may be more at risk for psychiatric and cognitive complications related to cannabis use. As states continue to implement changes in cannabis laws, understanding specific state trends and how policies affect the rate and intensity of cannabis use among adolescents is essential.

The advantages of educating youth about the risks and adverse outcomes of smoking cannabis in health care settings and in the public domain are well known; however, further research is needed to ascertain the most efficacious way to deliver this information to youth.

Adolescent populations frequently face substantial hurdles to seeking medical help and prefer to seek assistance from nonprofessional sources, such as peers, and important adults in their lives, such as teachers and parents. These obstacles underscore the necessity for more research on the role of informal settings, such as schools, for prevention efforts.

SUMMARY

Increased cannabis use in adolescents has been linked to a variety of challenges in recent research. Although numerous national surveys reveal no substantial change in adolescent cannabis usage as a result of medical and recreational cannabis legalization in various states, these data have several caveats. Recreational legalization is still relatively new, so trends may not have surfaced or been detected. Monitoring national data for cannabis use has significant limitations, such as survey discrepancies and small sample sizes. As cannabis usage continues to evolve in the face of increasing legalization, the medical community will continue to observe adverse health impacts on youth.

Clinicians are uniquely poised to address the negative health impacts of adolescent cannabis use and have a critical role in not just universal screening and treatment but also prevention. Clinicians should share information on adverse outcomes, such as the dangers of driving after using cannabis, as well as different modes of delivery and potency. In some circumstances, engaging parents can be valuable; however, patient confidentiality and privacy are paramount, and parental involvement should be first discussed with the adolescent. Parents should be informed that their own cannabis or other substance-related behaviors may influence their adolescent's perceptions and usage levels. Clinicians and school staff should work in conjunction to focus attention on special populations at risk of increased usage. Some specific clinical guidelines can be found in Boxes 1 and 2.

CLINICS CARE POINTS

Talking with children/adolescents about cannabis use in cannabis-legal states

- It is critical that parents, medical providers, and educators know how to best mitigate the risks associated with easy access and increased use of cannabis among children and teens.

- Adults (including parents and clinicians) should be honest, listen, share the facts, and offer support when talking to teens about cannabis.

- Parents should discuss the health effects of cannabis use and the consequences of use.

- Parents should warn teens about the risks of using edibles and driving while high on cannabis.

- Parents can talk with children about an "exit plan" to avoid drug use, such as texting a code word to a family member.

- Educators, clinicians, and other personnel in contact with youth should bring the conversation about risk and health effects of cannabis into the mainstream.

To address adolescent substance use, schools should:

- Offer systematic and efficient ways of reaching a wider population of young people, including essential screening in school-based clinics.

- Offer screening, brief interventions, and referral to treatment in school-based health centers to detect those at risk of developing substance use problems and facilitate referrals for those who are likely dependent or experiencing problems associated with or worsened by a substance use disorder.[45]

- Eliminate zero tolerance policies and replace with policies more conducive to school retention and academic remediation.

DISCLOSURE

The author K. Ladegard has nothing to disclose. D. Bhatia was supported by a Post-doctoral training grant, Grant Number T32 MH015442.

REFERENCES

1. Chawla D, Yang YC, Desrosiers TA, et al. Past-month cannabis use among US individuals from 2002–2015: an age-period-cohort analysis. Drug Alcohol Depend 2018;193:177–82.
2. Chadi N, Levy S. What Every Pediatric Gynecologist should know about marijuana Use in adolescents. J Pediatr Adolesc Gynecol 2019;32(4):349–53. https://doi.org/10.1016/j.jpag.2019.03.004.
3. Volkow ND, Baler RD, Compton WM, et al. Adverse health effects of marijuana Use. N Engl J Med 2014;370(23):2219–27. https://doi.org/10.1056/NEJMra 1402309.
4. Cerdá M, Sarvet AL, Wall M, et al. Medical marijuana laws and adolescent use of marijuana and other substances: alcohol, cigarettes, prescription drugs, and other illicit drugs. Drug and Alcohol Dependence 2018;183:62–8. https://doi.org/10.1016/j.drugalcdep.2017.10.021.
5. Choo EK, Benz M, Zaller N, et al. The impact of state medical marijuana Legislation on adolescent marijuana Use. J Adolesc Health 2014;55(2):160–6. https://doi.org/10.1016/j.jadohealth.2014.02.018.

6. Smart R, Pacula RL. Early evidence of the impact of cannabis legalization on cannabis use, cannabis use disorder, and the use of other substances: findings from state policy evaluations. Am J Drug Alcohol Abuse 2019;45(6):644–63. https://doi.org/10.1080/00952990.2019.1669626.

7. Pacula RL, Powell D, Heaton P, et al. Assessing the effects of medical marijuana laws on marijuana Use: the Devil is in the Details: assessing the effects of medical marijuana laws. J Pol Anal Manage 2015;34(1):7–31. https://doi.org/10.1002/pam.21804.

8. Wen H, Hockenberry J, Cummings JR. The effect of medical marijuana laws on marijuana, alcohol, and hard drug Use. National Bureau of Economic Research 2014.

9. Thurstone C, Lieberman SA, Schmiege SJ. Medical marijuana diversion and associated problems in adolescent substance treatment. Drug and alcohol dependence 2011;118(2–3):489–92.

10. Brooks-Russell A, Ma M, Levinson AH, et al. Adolescent marijuana use, marijuana-related perceptions, and Use of other substances before and after initiation of retail marijuana sales in Colorado (2013–2015). Prev Sci 2019;20(2): 185–93. https://doi.org/10.1007/s11121-018-0933-2.

11. Cerdá M, Mauro C, Hamilton A, et al. Association between recreational marijuana legalization in the United States and changes in marijuana Use and cannabis Use disorder from 2008 to 2016. JAMA Psychiatry 2020;77(2):165. https://doi.org/10.1001/jamapsychiatry.2019.3254.

12. Anderson DM, Rees DI, Sabia JJ, et al. Association of marijuana legalization with marijuana Use among US high school students, 1993-2019. JAMA Netw Open 2021;4(9):e2124638. https://doi.org/10.1001/jamanetworkopen.2021.24638.

13. Substance Abuse and Mental Health Services Administration. (2018). Key substance use and mental health indicators in the United States: Results from the 2017 National Survey on Drug Use and Health (HHS Publication No. SMA 18-5068, NSDUH Series H-53). Rockville, MD: Center for Behavioral Health Statistics and Quality, Substance Abuse and Mental Health Services Administration. Retrieved from https://www.samhsa.gov/data/ Accessed on January 20, 2022.

14. Cerdá M, Wall M, Feng T, et al. Association of state recreational marijuana laws with adolescent marijuana Use. JAMA Pediatr 2017;171(2):142. https://doi.org/10.1001/jamapediatrics.2016.3624.

15. Fleming CB, Guttmannova K, Cambron C, et al. Examination of the divergence in trends for adolescent marijuana use and marijuana-specific risk factors in Washington State. J Adolesc Health 2016;59(3):269–75.

16. Miech RA, Johnston L, O'Malley PM, et al. Trends in use of marijuana and attitudes toward marijuana among youth before and after decriminalization: the case of California 2007–2013. Int J Drug Policy 2015;26(4):336–44.

17. Salas-Wright CP, Vaughn MG, Todic J, et al. Trends in the disapproval and use of marijuana among adolescents and young adults in the United States: 2002–2013. Am J Drug Alcohol Abuse 2015;41(5):392–404.

18. Schuermeyer J, Salomonsen-Sautel S, Price RK, et al. Temporal trends in marijuana attitudes, availability and use in Colorado compared to non-medical marijuana states: 2003–11. Drug and alcohol dependence 2014;140:145–55.

19. Martins SS, Mauro CM, Santaella-Tenorio J, et al. State-level medical marijuana laws, marijuana use and perceived availability of marijuana among the general US population. Drug and alcohol dependence 2016;169:26–32.

20. Schulenberg JE, Johnston LD, O'Malley PM, Bachman JG, Miech RA, Patrick ME. Monitoring the future national survey results on drug use, 1975-2016: Volume II, college students and adults ages 19-55. Published online 2017.

21. Johnston LD, O'Malley PM, Bachman JG, et al. Monitoring the Future national survey results on drug use, 1975-2013: Volume I, Secondary school students. Published online 2014.

22. Bailey C, Pearson E. Development and trial of an educational tool to support the accessibility evaluation process. In: Proceedings of the International cross-disciplinary Conference on Web accessibility - W4A '11. ACM Press 2011;1. https://doi.org/10.1145/1969289.1969293.

23. Kosterman R, Bailey JA, Guttmannova K, et al. Marijuana legalization and parents' attitudes, use, and parenting in Washington State. J Adolesc Health 2016; 59(4):450–6.

24. Bull SS, Brooks-Russell A, Davis JM, et al. Awareness, perception of risk and behaviors related to retail marijuana among a sample of Colorado youth. J Community Health 2017;42(2):278–86.

25. Wadsworth E, Craft S, Calder R, et al. Prevalence and use of cannabis products and routes of administration among youth and young adults in Canada and the United States: a systematic review. Addict Behav 2022;107258.

26. Smart R, Caulkins JP, Kilmer B, et al. Variation in cannabis potency and prices in a newly legal market: evidence from 30 million cannabis sales in Washington state: legal cannabis potency and price variation. Addiction 2017;112(12): 2167–77. https://doi.org/10.1111/add.13886.

27. Hall W, Lynskey M. Assessing the public health impacts of legalizing recreational cannabis use: the US experience. World Psychiatry 2020;19(2):179–86. https://doi.org/10.1002/wps.20735.

28. Chandra S, Radwan MM, Majumdar CG, et al. New trends in cannabis potency in USA and Europe during the last decade (2008–2017). Eur Arch Psychiatry Clin Neurosci 2019;269(1):5–15.

29. Morean ME, Kong G, Camenga DR, et al. High school students' use of electronic cigarettes to vaporize cannabis. Pediatrics 2015;136(4):611–6.

30. Bell C, Slim J, Flaten HK, et al. Butane hash oil Burns associated with marijuana liberalization in Colorado. J Med Toxicol 2015;11(4):422–5. https://doi.org/10.1007/s13181-015-0501-0.

31. Keller CJ, Chen EC, Brodsky K, et al. A case of butane hash oil (marijuana wax)–induced psychosis. Substance Abuse 2016;37(3):384–6. https://doi.org/10.1080/08897077.2016.1141153.

32. Rickner SS, Cao D, Kleinschmidt K, et al. A little "dab" will do ya' in: a case report of neuro-and cardiotoxicity following use of cannabis concentrates. Clin Toxicol 2017;55(9):1011–3. https://doi.org/10.1080/15563650.2017.1334914.

33. Borodovsky JT, Lee DC, Crosier BS, et al. U.S. cannabis legalization and use of vaping and edible products among youth. Drug and Alcohol Dependence 2017; 177:299–306. https://doi.org/10.1016/j.drugalcdep.2017.02.017.

34. Nicksic NE, Do EK, Barnes AJ. Cannabis legalization, tobacco prevention policies, and Cannabis use in E-cigarettes among youth. Drug and Alcohol Dependence 2020;206:107730. https://doi.org/10.1016/j.drugalcdep.2019.107730.

35. Goodwin RD, Pacek LR, Copeland J, et al. Trends in daily cannabis use among cigarette smokers: United States, 2002–2014. Am J Public Health 2018;108(1): 137–42.

36. Masonbrink AR, Richardson T, Hall M, et al. Trends in adolescent cannabis-related hospitalizations by state legalization laws, 2008–2019. J Adolesc Health 2021;69(6):999–1005.

37. Castellanos-Ryan N, Pingault JB, Parent S, et al. Adolescent cannabis use, change in neurocognitive function, and high-school graduation: a longitudinal study from early adolescence to young adulthood. Development psychopathology 2017;29(4):1253–66.

38. Mashhoon Y, Sagar KA, Gruber SA. Cannabis use and consequences. Pediatr Clin 2019;66(6):1075–86.

39. Meier MH, Caspi A, Ambler A, et al. Persistent cannabis users show neuropsychological decline from childhood to midlife. Proc Natl Acad Sci 2012;109(40): E2657–64. https://doi.org/10.1073/pnas.1206820109.

40. Lisdahl KM. Dare to delay? The impacts of adolescent alcohol and marijuana use onset on cognition, brain structure, and function. Front Psychiatry 2013;4:53.

41. Silins E, Horwood LJ, Patton GC, et al. Young adult sequelae of adolescent cannabis use: an integrative analysis. Lancet Psychiatry 2014;1(4):286–93.

42. Smart Approaches to marijuana. Lessons learned from marijuana Legalization In four U.S. States and D.C. Smart Approaches to Marijuana; 2021.

43. Colorado department of public health and environment. Healthy Kids Colorado survey. 2018. Available at: https://cdphe.colorado.gov/healthy-kids-colorado-survey-data-tables-and-reports. Accessed January 6, 2022.

44. Evans-Whipp TJ, Plenty SM, Catalano RF, et al. Longitudinal effects of school drug policies on student marijuana use in Washington State and Victoria, Australia. Am J Public Health 2015;105(5):994–1000.

45. Nunes AP, Richmond MK, Marzano K, et al. Ten years of implementing screening, brief intervention, and referral to treatment (SBIRT): Lessons learned. Substance abuse 2017;38(4):508–12.

46. Levine A, Clemenza K, Rynn M, et al. Evidence for the risks and consequences of adolescent cannabis exposure. J Am Acad Child Adolesc Psychiatry 2017;56(3): 214–25.

47. Toni Heron MBBS DM, Roger Gibson M, Wendel Abel MBBS DM. Gender and suicidal behaviour among adolescents who use alcohol. Int Public Health J 2017;9(1):51.

48. Borges G, Bagge CL, Orozco R. A literature review and meta-analyses of cannabis use and suicidality. J Affective Disord 2016;195:63–74.

49. Doucette ML, Borrup KT, Lapidus G, et al. Effect of Washington State and Colorado's cannabis legalization on death by suicides. Prev Med 2021;148:106548.

50. Gobbi G, Atkin T, Zytynski T, et al. Association of cannabis use in adolescence and risk of depression, anxiety, and suicidality in young adulthood: a systematic review and meta-analysis. JAMA psychiatry 2019;76(4):426–34.

51. Coffey C, Patton GC. Cannabis use in adolescence and young adulthood: a review of findings from the Victorian Adolescent Health Cohort Study. Can J Psychiatry 2016;61(6):318–27.

52. Fergusson DM, Boden JM, Horwood LJ. Psychosocial sequelae of cannabis use and implications for policy: findings from the Christchurch Health and Development Study. Social Psychiatry Psychiatr Epidemiol 2015;50(9):1317–26.

53. Nocon A, Wittchen HU, Pfister H, et al. Dependence symptoms in young cannabis users? A prospective epidemiological study. J Psychiatr Res 2006; 40(5):394–403.

54. Silins E, Swift W, Slade T, et al. A prospective study of the substance use and mental health outcomes of young adult former and current cannabis users. Drug alcohol Rev 2017;36(5):618–25.
55. Ogourtsova T, Kalaba M, Gelinas I, et al. Cannabis use and driving-related performance in young recreational users: a within-subject randomized clinical trial. CMAJ open 2018;6(4):E453.
56. Li L, Hu G, Schwebel DC, et al. Analysis of US teen driving after using marijuana, 2017. JAMA Netw Open 2020;3(12):e2030473.
57. Wang GS, Davies SD, Halmo LS, et al. Impact of marijuana legalization in Colorado on adolescent emergency and urgent care visits. J Adolesc Health 2018; 63(2):239–41.
58. Delva-Clark H, Wang GS, Ryall KA, et al. Adolescent marijuana exposures reported to the Rocky Mountain Poison Center. In: clinical toxicology58. MILTON PARK: TAYLOR & FRANCIS LTD 2-4 PARK SQUARE; 2020. p. 1117–8. ABINGDON OR14 4RN, OXON.
59. Levy SJ, Williams JF. Committee on Substance Use and Prevention. Substance use screening, brief intervention, and referral to treatment. Pediatrics 2016; 138(1):e20161211.
60. Hall KE, Monte AA, Chang T, et al. Mental health–related emergency department visits associated with cannabis in Colorado. Acad Emerg Med 2018;25(5): 526–37.
61. Hopfer C. Implications of marijuana legalization for adolescent substance use. Substance abuse 2014;35(4):331–5.
62. Sevigny EL. The effects of medical marijuana laws on cannabis-involved driving. Accid Anal Prev 2018;118:57–65.
63. Tefft BC, Arnold LS, Grabowski JG. Prevalence of marijuana involvement in fatal crashes: Washington, 2010–2014. Published online 2016.
64. Kim HS, Anderson JD, Saghafi O, et al. Cyclic vomiting presentations following marijuana liberalization in Colorado. Acad Emerg Med 2015;22(6):694–9.
65. Wang GS, Buttorff C, Wilks A, et al. Changes in emergency department encounters for vomiting after cannabis legalization in Colorado. JAMA Netw open 2021; 4(9):e2125063.
66. Firth CL, Hajat A, Dilley JA, et al. Implications of cannabis legalization on juvenile justice outcomes and racial disparities. Am J Prev Med 2020;58(4):562–9.
67. Firth CL, Davenport S, Smart R, et al. How high: differences in the developments of cannabis markets in two legalized states. Int J Drug Pol 2020;75:102611.
68. Plunk AD, Peglow SL, Harrell PT, et al. Youth and adult arrests for cannabis possession after decriminalization and legalization of cannabis. JAMA Pediatr 2019;173(8):763–9.
69. Dickson B, Mansfield C, Guiahi M, et al. Recommendations from cannabis dispensaries about first-trimester cannabis use. Obstet Gynecol 2018;131(6):1031.
70. Rodriguez CE, Sheeder J, Allshouse AA, et al. Marijuana use in young mothers and adverse pregnancy outcomes: a retrospective cohort study. BJOG: An Int J Obstet Gynaecol 2019;126(12):1491–7.
71. Gunn JKL, Rosales CB, Center KE, et al. Prenatal exposure to cannabis and maternal and child health outcomes: a systematic review and meta-analysis. BMJ open 2016;6(4):e009986.
72. Hayatbakhsh MR, Flenady VJ, Gibbons KS, et al. Birth outcomes associated with cannabis use before and during pregnancy. Pediatr Res 2012;71(2):215–9.
73. Scheyer AF, Melis M, Trezza V, et al. Consequences of perinatal cannabis exposure. Trends Neurosciences 2019;42(12):871–84.

Cannabis Use Disorder in Adolescents

Daniel Hashemi, MD[a],*, Kevin Gray, MD[b]

KEYWORDS

• Adolescent • Youth • Marijuana • Cannabis use disorder

KEY POINTS

- Adolescence is a particularly important time for cognitive/neurologic growth.
- The endocannabinoid system is involved in multiple hormonal and neurologic processes. Endogenous cannabinoid receptor 1 (CB1) receptors play a major role in regulating the rapid development of the prefrontal cortex and other areas of the developing brain important for cognition, memory, and mood. Exogenous introduction of delta-9-tetrahydrocannabinol, which binds to CB1, may alter this development and play a role in known chronic adverse effects on cognition, psychiatric health, and psychosocial outcomes.
- Adverse effects of cannabis use (cognitive, psychosocial, psychiatric, physical) are generally more pronounced in those who start using at a young age.
- Recent trends toward increased potency of cannabis and lower perceived risk of use among adolescents increase the importance of psychoeducation, prevention, and treatment.
- Cannabis use generally reaches the definition of becoming a use disorder if a patient displays continued use despite negative consequences.

INTRODUCTION

With increasing amounts of information and misinformation regarding cannabis available to the public, it is becoming increasingly important for clinicians working with adolescents to have a strong scientific foundation on how cannabis use can affect young patients. Adolescence is a particularly important period in life. Adolescents' brains undergo significant changes, including but not limited to, synaptic pruning, myelination, and development of the prefrontal cortex. The endocannabinoid system is spread widely throughout the central nervous system and plays an important role in multiple important physiologic processes, including neural development, psychiatric disease, sleep-wake

This article originally appeared in *Child and Adolescent Psychiatric Clinics*, Volume 32 Issue 1, January 2023.

[a] Department of Psychiatry and Behavioral Sciences, Medical University of South Carolina, 67 President Street, Charleston, South Carolina 29425, USA; [b] Medical University of South Carolina, 125 Doughty Street, Suite 190, Charleston, SC 29425, USA

* Corresponding author.

E-mail address: hashemid@musc.edu

https://doi.org/10.1016/j.psc.2023.03.013
0193-953X/23/© 2023 Elsevier Inc. All rights reserved.

psych.theclinics.com

cycle regulation, inflammation, and appetite. Most importantly for adolescents, the endocannabinoid system plays an important role in regulating the development of the prefrontal cortex and other key brain regions during this period of rapid development.[1] The cannabinoid receptor 1 (CB1) is concentrated in the prefrontal cortex, hippocampus, and amygdala, regions of the brain that play an important regulatory role in executive function, memory, mood, and anxiety. Exogenous disruption of this system via exposure to delta-9-tetrahydrocannabinol (THC), the psychoactive component of cannabis, has been shown to alter the developing brain in both animal and human studies.[2]

Because of cannabis' psychoactive role, the importance of adolescent brain development, and trends of increasing potency of cannabis, it is important for clinicians working in both pediatric primary care and behavioral health clinical settings to have up-to-date scientific knowledge on the impact of cannabis use disorder in adolescents. This article focuses on trends in adolescent cannabis use, changes in public perception, cannabis' acute and chronic physiologic effects, the definition of cannabis use disorder, and associations with cannabis use disorder.

EPIDEMIOLOGY OF USE

Cannabis is the most commonly used illicit substance among adolescents in the United States. In 2020, it is estimated 43.7% of US 12th graders had tried cannabis in their lifetime. The prevalence of 12th graders having used in the past year has hovered in the mid 30% over the past decade, most recently, 35.2% in 2020. Approximately one in 15 12th graders (6.9%) used daily or nearly daily. Daily use, a pattern most associated with developing a use disorder, has increased significantly (from approximately 2%) over the past 30 years.[3] Seventeen percent of adolescents who try cannabis will develop a use disorder, which is nearly double the rate of adults who try cannabis.[4]

Cannabis' potency and variety of methods of use have increased dramatically over the past 2 decades. THC is the primary psychoactive component of cannabis. As such, it is concerning that THC concentrations have increased dramatically from 8.9% in 2008 to 17.1% in 2017. In addition to increased potency, legalization and commercialization of cannabis have been associated with a significant increase in alternative methods of use, including vaping, edibles, capsules, creams, and synthetics. Moreover, alternative methods of using cannabis (oils, concentrates) have shown an even more dramatic increase in the rate of THC potency (6.7% to 55.7%).[5] Butane hash oil, colloquially referred to as dabs, wax, or shatter, can achieve higher THC concentrations than plant-based cannabis through manufactural techniques.[6] The percentage of 12th graders who have vaped marijuana, which tends to have these higher concentrations, has been steadily increasing from over the past 4 years from 9.5% in 2017 to 22.1% in 2020.[3]

Synthetic cannabinoids (also referred to as "Spice" or "K2") are less commonly used than cannabis. However, synthetics are still prevalent with 2.4% of 12th graders having used them in the past year in 2020, down from a peak of nearly 12% in 2012.[3] Synthetics have a wide variety of potency, have higher binding affinity for CB1 and CB2 receptors, and are often mixed with other illicit substances. Because of increased affinity, the unpredictability of potency, and potential cross-contamination, synthetics are associated with more severe adverse effects.

PUBLIC PERCEPTION

The public has been inundated with information and misinformation regarding reported effects, both positive and negative, of cannabis. As such, pediatric primary care and behavioral health clinicians can play an important role by providing psycho-education to patients and families via accurate information and recommendations.

The past 2 decades have also seen drastic changes in legal policies regarding cannabis use, both recreationally and medicinally (detailed in other articles). These legal changes have been associated with a societal decline in the perceived risk of cannabis use in adolescents. In 2019, only 30.5% of adolescents saw regular cannabis use as a great risk compared to 77.9% of adolescents in 1989.[3] It is important to note that despite increased state-level legalization and availability via dispensaries, there is no Food and Drug Administration regulation of commercial cannabinoid products. This has led to cases of inaccurate labeling (eg, products labeled as "CBD only" found to have THC, products geared toward specific symptoms despite lack of evidence), which can influence public perception and use patterns.

There is an inverse relationship between perception of risk and cannabis use.[7] Given this relationship as well as the risks of misinformation, it is important that clinicians working with this population have scientifically accurate information regarding risks of use and treatment recommendations.

PHYSIOLOGIC EFFECTS
Acute Effects

Acute intoxication of cannabis is variable among users, although the "high" of ingestion can include euphoria, increased bonding with peers, and occasionally pleasant perceptual disturbances. Smoked effects begin almost immediately and typically last 2 to 3 hours, whereas alternative methods are more variable but typically take longer to have an effect.[8,9]

Common physiologic changes of cannabis use include tachycardia, dry mouth, and conjunctival/scleral injection. Respiratory symptoms (wheezing, coughing) can occur as well, with higher rates associated with vaping.[10]

Supporting the importance of the endocannabinoid system's impact on the brain, cannabis use is associated with short-term neurologic and psychiatric effects. Neurologic effects include short-term impairments in memory, judgment, cognition, coordination, and balance. Given cannabis' impact on perceptual disturbances, judgment, and coordination, it is not surprising cannabis use is also associated with an increased risk of motor vehicle collisions.[4] Short-term psychiatric symptoms can include anxiety, paranoia, and hallucinations. Cannabis use is associated with increased suicidality (increased incidence of suicidal ideation, suicide attempts, and suicide completion).[11] In a study in Colorado in 2016, cannabis became the most common substance present in toxicology of adolescents who died by suicide.[12]

Treatment of acute intoxication is supportive. Given potential increased risk for suicide, assessing for safety in acutely intoxicated patients is vital. In patients experiencing psychotic symptoms, both gathering collateral information and observation may be helpful to elucidate the chronicity of symptoms and diagnostic clarity.

Withdrawal

Approximately one-third of regular users experience cannabis withdrawal, whereas heavy users are even more likely (50%–95%) to experience withdrawal.[7] The rate of cannabis withdrawal is likely underestimated by both the public and professionals. However, withdrawal is important to recognize given its association with difficulty quitting and frequent use of cannabis to relieve withdrawal symptoms. The symptoms of cannabis withdrawal likely play a role in some patients' belief that cannabis helps with anxiety, as the use of cannabis while withdrawing can reduce the effects of withdrawal.

Cannabis withdrawal symptoms vary depending on individual factors as well as quantity/frequency of use. Symptoms can include depression, anxiety, irritability, aggression, weight loss, and decreased appetite.

Cannabis withdrawal syndrome is defined as 3 or more of the following[13]:

- Anxiety and/or restlessness
- Depression and/or irritability
- Insomnia or odd dreams
- Physical symptoms, such as tremors
- Decreased appetite

Cannabis withdrawal can last 1 day to 2 weeks. There is currently no pharmacologic treatment for cannabis withdrawal; however, cognitive and behavioral skills and support can help patients experiencing withdrawal. Helpful behavioral techniques (detailed further in other articles) can include urge surfing, distraction, engaging in non-drug-related activities, and encouraging healthy social support. As such, it is important for clinicians to have discussions with patients and families regarding symptom expectations, timelines, and healthy coping skills.

Chronic effects

Cannabis use is associated with chronic cognitive, psychosocial, psychiatric, and physical adverse effects. Many studies show the effects of use are more severe in those who start cannabis use at a younger age.[4]

Associated cognitive outcomes include lower IQ; however, it is unclear if this relationship is causal.[4,14] Cannabis use is also associated with negative psychosocial outcomes, including higher rates of life dissatisfaction and school dropout. Earlier use is associated with lower income, higher rates of unemployment, and higher rates of criminal behavior.[15,16]

Regarding psychiatric comorbidities, cannabis use is associated with higher rates of psychosis. It is debated whether this relationship is causal, although some studies do support a pathway from cannabis use to psychosis and not the reverse.[17] Daily cannabis use, younger age of onset of use, and higher THC potency are associated with developing a psychotic episode, which is particularly concerning given increasing THC concentration in cannabis preparations (detailed in the section Epidemiology of Use). In addition to psychosis, cannabis use is associated with higher rates of other substance use disorders (including alcohol and tobacco/nicotine), major depressive disorder, generalized anxiety disorder, attention-deficit hyperactivity disorder, posttraumatic stress disorder, conduct disorder, multiple personality disorders,[18] new-onset manic symptoms,[19] and suicide attempts.[20]

In addition to cognitive and psychiatric effects, chronic cannabis use has physical adverse effects, including cannabinoid hyperemesis syndrome[21] as well as lung injury, particularly in those who use cannabis via vaping or using e-cigarettes.[22]

CANNABIS USE DISORDER AND SEVERITY

The *Diagnostic and Statistical Manual (DSM)* of Mental Health Disorders, fifth edition, defines Cannabis Use Disorder with the following criteria[23]:

Use of cannabis for at least 1 year with the presence of 2 or more of the following symptoms, accompanied by significant impairment of functioning and distress:

- Difficulty containing the use of cannabis. "Have you used more than you had planned to use?"

- Failed efforts to discontinue and/or reduce use. "Have you tried to quit or cut back but felt like you couldn't stick with it?"
- An inordinate amount of time spent acquiring/using cannabis or recovering from the effects of cannabis.
- Cravings or desires to use cannabis (including intrusive thoughts, images, dreams, and perceptions).
- Continued use of cannabis despite adverse consequences, including criminal charges, ultimatums of abandonment from family/friends/partners, and poor productivity.
- The desire to use cannabis takes priority over other important activities in life, such as school, work, hygiene, and other responsibilities.
- Cannabis is used in contexts that are potentially dangerous, such as operating a motor vehicle.
- Continued use of cannabis despite awareness of physical and/or psychological problems attributed to use.
- Tolerance to cannabis, defined as either a larger amount of cannabis needed to obtain the psychoactive effect experienced when use first began or reduced effect of use from the same amount of cannabis
- Withdrawal symptoms (described in detail above) or use of cannabis or a similar substance to prevent withdrawal.

Cannabis use disorder can be further specified as mild (2–3 of the above criteria), moderate (4–5 of the criteria), or severe (6 or more criteria). Increasing severity of cannabis use disorder is associated with worse mental health and psychosocial outcomes (detailed above in the section Chronic Effects). In addition, earlier age of onset of cannabis use is associated with higher rates of developing into use disorder, making prevention and treatment of adolescents particularly important. If a clinician is concerned for cannabis use disorder, it is beneficial to screen for all substance use disorders given high rates of cooccurrence. All substance use disorder criteria have the same symptoms detailed above for cannabis.

Cannabis use disorder is considered to be in early remission if the above criteria were previously met less than 12 months ago but greater than 3 months ago. Cannabis use disorder is considered to be in sustained remission if the above criteria were last met greater than 12 months ago.

As detailed in the *DSM*, cannabis use disorder is a clinical diagnosis and does not depend on drug screens. However, urine drug testing is considered an important component of cannabis use disorder treatment, as it provides an objective marker of goal behavior change (abstinence or not). Drug tests (most commonly via urine testing) typically test for THC, a common cannabis metabolite, with a common cutoff of 50 ng/mL. Drug screens typically test use in the few days before the test, although frequent heavy users may test positive for longer. Synthetic cannabis and other derivatives can test negative, even in recent use, given different structural compositions. Drug screens should not be depended upon as a sole source of information, particularly as providers are establishing clinical rapport and trust. Qualitative (positive or negative) drug screens are also less helpful in those patients who are in the process of reducing use rather than abstaining completely.

Treatment of cannabis use disorder is detailed in a further article.

ASSOCIATIONS WITH CANNABIS USE DISORDER

Notable associations with developing cannabis use disorder include the following[18,20]:

- Male sex
- Early onset of use
- Other use disorders
- Family history of use disorder
- History of tobacco use
- Lower socioeconomic status
- Family members who use cannabis
- Poor academic performance
- Unstable/abusive family
- Psychiatric diagnoses (major depressive disorder, generalized anxiety disorder, attention-deficit hyperactivity disorder, posttraumatic stress disorder, conduct disorder)

IMPLICATIONS FOR CLINICAL PRACTICE

Pediatric primary care and behavioral health clinicians who work with adolescents play an important role in recognizing adolescent cannabis use, screening for cannabis use disorder, and educating patients/families on the risks of cannabis use on the developing adolescent brain. Providing accurate psychoeducation is increasingly important in an era of misinformation, increasing cannabis potency, and an ever-changing legal landscape.

CLINICS CARE POINTS

- There is an inverse relationship between perception of risk and cannabis use, making psychoeducation a valuable tool for both prevention and treatment of cannabis use disorder.
- With increasing numbers of alternative cannabinoid products and methods of cannabis use, it is important to assess patients' use pattern in order to tailor discussion of potential risks.
- When a diagnosis of cannabis use disorder has been met, clinicians should screen for commonly associated disorders, including other substance use disorders and psychiatric diagnoses (major depressive disorder, generalized anxiety disorder, attention-deficit hyperactivity disorder, posttraumatic stress disorder, conduct disorder, , conduct disorder).
- Cannabis withdrawal is common and can be a barrier to cessation or reduction of use. Clinicians should be prepared to discuss potential withdrawal symptoms, provide expectations regarding timeline of symptoms, and encourage behavioral techniques to assist patients who may experience withdrawal.

FUNDING SOURCES

R25DA020537, R01DA042114, R01DA042114.

REFERENCES

1. Meyer HC, Lee FS, Gee DG. The role of the endocannabinoid system and genetic variation in adolescent brain development. Neuropsychopharmacology 2017; 43(1):21–33.
2. Batalla A, Bhattacharyya S, Yücel M, et al. Structural and functional imaging studies in chronic cannabis users: a systematic review of adolescent and adult findings. PLoS One 2013;8(2):e55821.
3. Johnston LD, Miech RA, O'Malley PM, et al., "Monitoring the future national survey results on drug use, 1975 - 2020: volume i, secondary students." Monit Future.

Available at: www.monitoringthefuture.org//pubs/monographs/mtf-overview2020. pdf. Accessed October 30, 2021.

4. Volkow ND, Baler RD, Compton WM, et al. Adverse health effects of marijuana use. N Engl J Med 2014;370:2219–27.

5. Chandra S, Radwan MM, Majumdar CG, et al. New trends in cannabis potency in USA and Europe during the last decade (2008-2017). Eur Arch Psychiatry Clin Neurosci 2019;269(1):5–15.

6. Al-Zouabi I, Stogner JM, Miller BL, et al. Butane hash oil and dabbing: insights into use, amateur production techniques, and potential harm mitigation. Subst Abuse Rehabil 2018;9:91–101. https://doi.org/10.2147/SAR.S135252.

7. Hasin DS. US epidemiology of cannabis use and associated problems. Neuropsychopharmacology 2018;43(1):195–212.

8. Huestis MA, Smith ML. Cannabinoid markers in biological fluids and tissues: revealing intake. Trends Mol Med 2018;24(2):156–72.

9. Poyatos L, Pérez-Acevedo AP, Papaseit E, et al. Oral administration of cannabis and delta-9-tetrahydrocannabinol (THC) preparations: a systematic review. Medicine (Kaunas) 2020;56(6):309.

10. Boyd CJ, McCabe SE, Evans-Police RJ, et al. Cannabis, vaping, and respiratory symptoms in a probability sample of U.S. youth. J Adolesc Health 2021;69(1): 149–52.

11. Han B, Compton WM, Einstein EB, et al. Associations of suicidality trends with cannabis use as a function of sex and depression status. JAMA Netw Open 2021;4(6):e2113025.

12. Roberts BA. Legalized cannabis in Colorado emergency departments: a cautionary review of negative health and safety effects. West J Emerg Med 2019;20(4):557–72.

13. Gorelick DA, Levin KH, Copersino ML, et al. Diagnostic criteria for cannabis withdrawal syndrome. Drug Alcohol Depend 2012;123(1–3):141–7.

14. Meier MH, Caspi A, Ambler A, et al. Persistent cannabis users show neuropsychological decline from childhood to midlife. Proc Natl Acad Sci 2012;109(40): E2657–64. https://doi.org/10.1073/pnas.1206820109.

15. Fergusson DM, Boden JM. Cannabis use and later life outcomes. Addiction 2008; 103(6):969–76. https://doi.org/10.1111/j.1360-0443.2008.02221.x.

16. Brook JS, Lee JY, Finch SJ, et al. Adult work commitment, financial stability, and social environment as related to trajectories of marijuana use beginning in adolescence. Substance Abuse 2013;34(3):298–305. https://doi.org/10.1080/08897077.2013.775092.

17. Fergusson DM, Boden JM, Horwood LJ. Psychosocial sequelae of cannabis use and policy implications: findings from the Christchurch Health and Development Study. Soc Psychiatry Psychiatr Epidemiol 2015;50(9):1317–26. https://doi.org/10.1007/s00127-015-1070-x.

18. Hasin DS, Kerridge BT, Saha TD, et al. Prevalence and correlates of DSM-5 cannabis use disorder, 2012–2013: findings from the National Epidemiologic Survey on alcohol and related conditions–III. Am J Psychiatry 2016;173(6):588–99. https://doi.org/10.1176/appi.ajp.2015.15070907.

19. Gibbs M, Winsper C, Marwaha S, et al. Cannabis use and mania symptoms: a systematic review and meta-analysis. J Affect Disord 2015;171:39–47.

20. Silins E, Horwood LJ, Patton GC, et al. Young adult sequelae of adolescent cannabis use: an integrative analysis. Lancet Psychiatry 2014;1(4):286–93.

21. Sorensen CJ, DeSanto K, Borgelt L, et al. Cannabinoid hyperemesis syndrome: diagnosis, pathophysiology, and treatment-a systematic review. J Med Toxicol 2017;13(1):71–87.
22. Perrine CG, Pickens CM, Boehmer TK, et al. Characteristics of a multistate outbreak of lung injury associated with e-cigarette use, or vaping - the United States, 2019. MMWR Morb Mortal Wkly Rep 2019;68(39):860–4.
23. American Psychiatric Association. Diagnostic and Statistical Manual of Mental Disorders: DSM-5. Washington, DC: American Psychiatric Association; 2013.

Impact of Adolescent Cannabis Use on Neurocognitive and Brain Development

J. Cobb Scott, PhD[a,b,*]

KEYWORDS

- Cannabis • Marijuana • Adolescence • Neuropsychological functioning • Memory
- Brain development

KEY POINTS

- Converging evidence indicates that ongoing, frequent cannabis use in adolescence is associated with small reductions in neurocognitive functioning.
- Abstinence from cannabis is likely to lead to some recovery in cognitive functioning in adolescents.
- Adolescent-onset, sustained, long-term use of cannabis may result in cognitive deficits that do not recover as readily with abstinence.
- There is some evidence that cannabis use in adolescence is associated with differences in brain structure, but these findings need replication.

INTRODUCTION

There have been substantial shifts in policy and perceptions regarding cannabis use in recent years. In 2018, cannabis was legalized in Canada for individuals 18 years and older. In the United States, cannabis has been legalized for adult recreational use in 18 states and for medical use in 37 states to date. Similar movements toward cannabis

This article originally appeared in *Child and Adolescent Psychiatric Clinics*, Volume 32 Issue 1, January 2023.

Conflicts of interest: The author declares no potential conflicts of interest. The views expressed in this article are those of the author and do not necessarily reflect the position or policy of the Department of Veterans Affairs.

[a] Department of Psychiatry, Perelman School of Medicine, University of Pennsylvania, 3700 Hamilton Walk, 5th Floor, Philadelphia, PA 19104, USA; [b] VISN4 Mental Illness Research, Education, and Clinical Center at the Corporal Michael J. Crescenz VA Medical Center, Philadelphia, PA 19104, USA

* Richards Building, 5th Floor, Suite 5A 3700 Hamilton Walk, Philadelphia, PA 19104-6085.

E-mail address: scott1@pennmedicine.upenn.edu

Twitter: @jcobbscott (J.C.S.)

legalization and decriminalization have occurred in Europe and Latin America. Concurrent with these trends, societal acceptance of cannabis use has increased, while the perception of its harms has decreased.[1] In 2020, 35% of US youth in 12th grade reported cannabis use in the past year, with 6.9% reporting daily or almost daily use.[2] While data indicate that the prevalence of cannabis use among adolescents and young adults has not reliably increased since 2010, daily use has increased in this population.[2,3] At the same time, the availability of cannabis in different forms such as concentrates, oils, and edibles has increased, and the levels of Δ^9-tetrahydrocannabinol (THC), the primary psychoactive ingredient in cannabis, have increased in both flower and concentrate forms.[4,5] Given these changes in cannabis policy and use, there has been considerable interest in research examining health risks of cannabis use, especially in adolescence and young adulthood, when most substance initiation occurs.[6]

This review will summarize the current state of research on associations between adolescent cannabis use, neurocognitive functioning, and brain development. Throughout, the review focuses on a critical question of significant public health importance: are there heightened risks for cognitive and brain development associated with adolescent cannabis use? To address this question, the review first provides critical background information on the neural circuitry involved in cannabis use and the involvement of these systems in neurodevelopment. Next, integrative summaries of research into associations between cannabis use and cognitive functioning, brain structure, and brain functioning will be provided. These summaries will focus primarily on findings in individuals without significant psychopathology (eg, psychosis) or substance use comorbidity (eg, cocaine use), though comorbid mental health symptoms, alcohol use, and nicotine use are very common in these samples. Furthermore, where possible, this review will highlight findings from large, representative studies; meta-analyses; twin and family studies; and longitudinal studies. As discussed below, cross-sectional studies with small, selective samples are more likely to lead to imprecise estimates of any potential true effect, resulting in lower replicability of findings and the potential for both false positive and false negative results,[7] especially with the smaller effect sizes expected in neuroimaging and neuropsychological research into cannabis use for example,.[8,9] Larger studies, meta-analyses, longitudinal research, and twin and family studies can minimize problems with reduced statistical power and help resolve discrepancies and confounds often encountered in smaller, cross-sectional studies. Finally, we conclude with an overview of findings, limitations of the current literature, future directions, and clinical care points related to this body of research.

Neurocircuitry of Cannabis

The psychoactive effects of cannabis are primarily driven by Δ^9-THC, one of at least 85 cannabinoids in *Cannabis sativa* discovered to date.[10] Cannabinoids bind with specific G-protein-coupled receptors known as cannabinoid receptors (CB-Rs). Two primary CB-Rs have been well characterized to date—CB_1 and CB_2. CB_1 receptors are primarily found in the central nervous system, with a high density in the basal ganglia, hippocampus, limbic system, and cerebellum.[11,12] CB_2 receptors are mainly found in peripheral tissue, particularly in the immune system. Endocannabinoids, such as anandamide and 2-arachidonoylglycerol, are naturally occurring ligands that activate CB-Rs. The endocannabinoids, CB-Rs, and enzymes responsible for the synthesis and degradation of endocannabinoids together comprise the endogenous (endocannabinoid [eCB]) system. CB_1 receptors in the brain have a wide role in maintaining neuronal inhibitory and excitatory balance via the regulation of neurotransmitter release and synaptic plasticity, especially glutamate and gamma-aminobutyric acid (GABA).[13] THC mimics endocannabinoids and primarily binds to CB_1 receptors in the brain, but its effects are more prolonged than those of endocannabinoids. Thus, THC seems to disrupt the regulatory roles of the eCB system and produces the behavioral, cognitive, memory, and motor effects of cannabis intoxication.

The eCB system is expressed early in brain development,[14] and animal and human studies suggest that the activity of endocannabinoids and CB-Rs may reach its peak during puberty.[15] Moreover, extensive research in the last 20 years has shown that the eCB system is critical to multiple neurodevelopmental processes from the early postnatal period through adolescence.[16,17] These processes include neuronal development and specification early in brain development, as well as neurogenesis, synaptic pruning, and white matter development during adolescence.[18,19] As such, the eCB system contributes to the development of efficient communication within and between brain networks during adolescence, including the establishment of adaptive cognitive functioning and emotion processing.

Adolescence as a Critical Neurodevelopmental Period

Adolescence is a period of dynamic neurobiological and behavioral changes. There are substantial increases in cognitive capacities, particularly in working memory, cognitive control, self-regulation, and abstraction.[20] Relatedly, marked neurodevelopmental changes occur during adolescence, including increased myelination, synaptic pruning, and increases in white matter development, with notable maturation of prefrontal regions and associated neural circuitry that proceeds into the mid-20s.[21–23] Because of this prolonged neurodevelopmental period, and the potential involvement of the endocannabinoid system in such brain-behavior changes, concerns have been raised regarding whether the use of cannabis during this "critical period" may disrupt normal trajectories of brain, emotional, and cognitive development.[15,24,25]

Preclinical studies have supported the biological plausibility of this hypothesis. Rodents at ages approximating adolescence have shown specific vulnerabilities to repeated exposure to THC or CB-R agonists compared with adult rodents.[26,27] Such studies have shown behavioral deficits in working memory and learning, reduced activity at synapses, and structural changes in the hippocampus with cannabinoid administration during adolescence, while few deficits appear with administration during periods approximating adulthood in rodents.[28,29] Interestingly, studies have shown some of these deficits to be reversible after short periods of abstinence.[30,31] Thus, evidence from animal models supports heightened adolescent vulnerability to cannabis exposure, with some behavioral deficits potentially reversible with abstinence.

Challenges of Evaluating Research Regarding Cannabis Use

Before reviewing the state of research on cannabis, cognitive functioning, and brain development, it is important to contextualize the challenges of research into the causal effects of cannabis use, as well as exposure research more broadly. Randomized controlled trials are the gold standard of evidence in determining causality. As randomized controlled trials of longer-term cannabis use are not feasible with adolescents because of legal, ethical, and safety concerns, studies examining the residual effects of cannabis are observational, and many use between-subject designs. Observational studies of exposures that individuals select, such as substance use, may create selection biases and present difficulty in removing the influence of confounding factors that may be associated both with the exposure and outcomes of interest. Such confounders have the potential to create spurious associations between cannabis and cognitive or brain outcomes, especially when effect sizes for exposure are modest.

For example, frequent cannabis users have been shown to have greater alcohol use, other substance use, and tobacco use[32]; personality traits that increase the risk for frequent substance use[33]; lower socioeconomic status[34]; higher trauma and adverse event exposure[35]; and more mental health comorbidities[36] than nonusers or occasional cannabis users. All of these factors have also been reported as associated with cognitive and brain development, and several are often difficult to resolve temporally in relation to cannabis use, including some that have been shown to predict cannabis initiation.[37] Alternatively, one could study cannabis users without these confounds to better isolate effects of cannabis, but the results are likely not generalizable to a typical population of frequent cannabis users (who are likely to have these other relevant factors), reducing the potential generalizability and impact of findings. Thus, studying cannabis in the "real world" and using proper frameworks and assumptions for modeling variables of interest is required. Without proper modeling of predictors, outcomes, and confounders, including the consideration of which variables should and should not be statistically controlled, it is challenging to rule out potential alternative explanations for findings and conduct effective causal inference.[38] Indeed, reducing the likelihood of alternative explanations for findings potentially caused by cannabis use will contribute to converging lines of evidence and inform public perception and policy related to cannabis.

As detailed below, there are also challenges in interpreting the published research on cannabis, cognitive functioning, and brain development due to substantial heterogeneity in methods, measurement, and sample characteristics. Continuous measures of cannabis use are rarely used due to difficulties in accurately measuring the amount or frequency of use (which is usually collected retrospectively), and heterogeneity is inevitably introduced by the different phenotypes (ie, operationalizations of grouping variables) used across studies. For example, studies of adolescent cannabis users have examined individuals diagnosed with a cannabis use disorder, daily cannabis users, regular cannabis users, those who have used cannabis a certain number of times, or those who initiated cannabis use before a particular age. There is likely to be substantial variability between and within these phenotypes in cannabis use frequency/intensity, as well as confounders, which may lead to noisy data. Furthermore, researchers sometimes explore more than one of these phenotypes as predictors but may only highlight the phenotype with significant findings. There are efforts underway to harmonize data collection related to cannabis,[39,40] but they have not been applied consistently to date. There are also persistent questions around variability in the selection, analysis, and reporting of neurocognitive data,[41,42] including publication bias, as well as analytical flexibility in neuroimaging studies.[43,44] Such "forking paths" are common in these studies and likely to affect the replicability of results.[45]

Highlighting the challenges in interpreting this line of research does not necessarily impede one's ability to come to informed conclusions about the risks of cannabis for cognitive and brain development. However, these data are complex, and it is beneficial to develop systematic approaches to interpretation, including the consideration of converging lines of replicable evidence. Readers should keep these critiques in mind when evaluating research in this area, including questions about variables of interest, measurement error, and causal conclusions.

RESIDUAL EFFECTS – COGNITIVE FUNCTIONING

Studies examining the relationship between cognitive functioning and problematic cannabis use in human adolescents have increased substantially over the past 2 decades. There is now a broad consensus that during acute cannabis intoxication, deficits in attention, executive functioning, and memory are evident,[46,47] though effects may differ for frequent cannabis users.[48,49] However, residual cognitive effects (ie, those persisting after episodes of acute intoxication) are still debated, especially after periods of abstinence from cannabis use.

There are several possible hypotheses regarding adolescent cannabis use and residual effects on cognitive functioning. The first is that cannabis use is associated with cognitive deficits that are caused by cannabis-associated neurotoxicity and are likely not reversible. If this hypothesis is true, abstinence from cannabis or reductions in cannabis use is unlikely to result in the amelioration of cognitive deficits. Of note, if this hypothesis is true, there are several additional questions regarding the dose of cannabis and timing of cannabis initiation that would be sufficient to cause such a decline. The second hypothesis is that cannabis is associated with cognitive deficits, but that these deficits are more associated with residual or withdrawal effects as opposed to neurotoxicity. If this hypothesis is true, cognitive deficits will be reversible with reductions in or abstinence from cannabis use. A third hypothesis is that any cognitive deficits observed in cannabis users are confounded by other correlated factors or due to preuse factors that would have caused deficits even in the absence of cannabis use. Of note, these hypotheses are not mutually exclusive, as deficits could be due to correlated or preuse factors *and* to cannabis itself, and some cognitive deficits may abate with abstinence while others persist.

Cross-Sectional Studies

Some of the early cross-sectional studies in adolescents and young adults reported relationships between heavy, frequent, or problematic cannabis use and poorer cognitive functioning, including executive functioning and reasoning, attention, speed of processing, and episodic learning and memory.[50–53] Relationships between earlier initiation of cannabis use and increased cognitive deficits were also reported.[54–56] Moreover, some studies showed dose-dependent effects of cannabis on cognitive functioning, such that individuals with more occasional use patterns (eg, once per week or less) display relatively intact cognitive functioning, while those with more frequent use or cannabis use disorders show impaired cognitive functioning.[51] However, most of these studies had small samples and were likely underpowered given the expected small-to-moderate cognitive effects associated with frequent cannabis use.[7]

Larger cross-sectional studies of community-based samples and meta-analyses have suggested greater complexity in findings related to cognitive functioning in adolescent cannabis users. For example, in a large community-based sample of adolescents and young adults (ages 14–21) from the Philadelphia Neurodevelopmental Cohort (PNC), Scott and colleagues[57] examined cognitive functioning in 227 past-year frequent cannabis users (2–3 times per week or more) and 940 past-year occasional cannabis users (1–2 times per week or less). Occasional cannabis users did not evidence cognitive deficits compared with nonusers and actually performed slightly better in certain cognitive domains. Moreover, the study found limited cognitive deficits in frequent cannabis users across the whole age range of the sample. However, they did find an interaction between age and cannabis use, such that frequent cannabis users at younger ages (14–17) performed worse in executive functioning than nonusers.

Meta-analyses quantitatively synthesize results of multiple studies and can estimate the magnitude of effect sizes (eg, cognitive test scores) and whether explanatory variables affect variability in outcomes across an existing literature. Meta-analyses can also address inconsistencies across a research literature by standardizing outcomes and reducing the impact of varying statistical power. One meta-analysis of cross-sectional studies examining cognitive functioning in adolescent and young adult cannabis users (up to age 26) has been conducted to date. This study found differences of a small magnitude (Cohen's d 0.21–0.33) between frequent cannabis users and nonusers in episodic learning and memory, executive functioning (cognitive flexibility, inhibition, and working memory), speed of processing, and attention.[9] These effect sizes and their relative magnitude across cognitive domains were similar to results from prior meta-analyses of adults.[58,59] However, several additional analyses highlighted the complexity of findings. First, neither age at first use nor the overall age of the sample in each study had a significant effect on the magnitude of the effect sizes. Second, studies of treatment-seeking individuals had larger magnitude of cognitive effects than studies of community samples. Finally, abstinence impacted the magnitude of effect sizes. Increasing length of abstinence—both the amount required by a study and the mean length reported by participants in a study—was associated with a smaller magnitude of effect sizes. In addition, studies that required an abstinence period from cannabis use of longer than 72 hours (corresponding to the postpeak period for most cannabis withdrawal symptoms[60]) had a very small, nonsignificant effect size. Together, these results support small reductions in specific neurocognitive domains with continuing cannabis use in adolescents and young adults but also raise uncertainty about the persistence of cannabis-associated cognitive alterations after periods of abstinence.

Longitudinal and Twin Studies

Cross-sectional research designs allow minimal causal inferences and cannot determine whether cognitive deficits were present before cannabis use or might be accounted for by other confounders. Unlike cross-sectional studies, longitudinal designs can examine trajectories of change and temporal relationships between variables of interest and may be able to explore whether preuse risk factors are distinct from the consequences of cannabis use. For instance, several studies have shown that adolescents at risk of developing problematic cannabis use display preuse cognitive vulnerabilities, such as deficits in working memory and inhibitory control,[61–64] which may place such individuals at greater risk of earlier and more frequent substance use[65–67] and confound interpretation of cognitive data. Consideration of such confounders is critical for the interpretation of observational longitudinal data.

Smaller longitudinal studies have linked continued cannabis use in adolescence to cognitive decline in processing speed, executive functions, and episodic memory.[61,68–70] However, similar to results from meta-analyses, deficits improve with verified abstinence over a period of weeks,[71,72] and cannabis abstinent adolescents and young adults often perform similarly to nonusers.[52,73–77]

Perhaps the strongest evidence for cannabis-associated cognitive deficits comes from analysis of the large Dunedin Longitudinal Study by Meier and colleagues.[78] In a landmark study of 1037 individuals followed from childhood to age 38, intelligent quotient (IQ) data were examined from individuals in childhood (before any cannabis use had occurred) and again at age 38. The authors showed that individuals who started using cannabis at least weekly by age 18 and continued using cannabis almost daily throughout early adulthood showed significant declines in IQ (especially on verbal IQ measures) between childhood and age 38, corresponding to approximately 6 IQ points. Moreover, individuals who used infrequently at age 38 still showed IQ decline if they used weekly before age 18, but those who did not initiate regular cannabis use before age 18 did not show decline if they had reduced their use by age 38. In other words, abstinence seemed to improve cognitive functioning in those who delayed the initiation of frequent cannabis use until after age 18. Of note, the authors found mostly similar results after adjusting for several other confounders, including other substance use, psychopathology, and recent cannabis use.

Additional work has extended these results in large cohort studies with longitudinal measurements of cognitive functioning. Mokrysz and colleagues[79] examined IQ data at age 15 after controlling for childhood IQ at age 8 in 2235 adolescents from the Avon Longitudinal Study of Parents and Children (ALSPAC). They found that cumulative cannabis use was negatively associated with IQ at age 15, and those who reported using cannabis 50 or more times had IQs that were almost 3 points lower than nonusers. However, when analyses controlled for several confounders, including adolescent cigarette, alcohol, and other substance use, any relationships between cumulative cannabis use and IQ were attenuated, indicating significant complexity in these relationships. In another study of 3232 individuals from the ALSPAC cohort, Mahedy and colleagues[80] found that early-onset regular cannabis use between ages 13 and 18 was associated with poorer working memory and response inhibition at age 24 compared with nonusers, even after controlling for socioeconomic status. However, analyses that attempted to examine causality in these relationships using Mendelian randomization[81] were inconclusive. Morin and colleagues[64] examined associations between cannabis, alcohol, and cognitive functioning in a unique dataset that repeatedly measured cognition and substance use between 7th and 10th grade in 3826 adolescents from Montreal, Canada. They used multilevel models to explore how changes in one variable (eg, cannabis use) were associated with changes in another (eg, working memory performance) over time by examining concurrent and time-lagged associations between variables. They found that the use of cannabis and alcohol were both associated with lower working memory, perceptual reasoning, and inhibitory control. Furthermore, they reported that cannabis was associated with episodic memory performance, but only transiently (potentially abating with abstinence). Finally, they found that cannabis use was associated with time-lagged effects on inhibitory control even after controlling for alcohol use. This finding was interpreted as potentially consistent with a neurotoxic effect of cannabis, though there was limited discussion of the magnitude of the effect or its potential clinical significance.

Several studies have taken advantage of informative cotwin control designs to help determine whether associations between cannabis use and cognitive functioning are confounded by genetic and family environment influences. In such studies, examining differences in cognitive functioning or decline between cannabis-exposed twins and their nonusing (or abstinent) siblings can help determine the feasibility of a causal association between cannabis use and cognitive functioning by accounting for unmeasured influences that are common for twin pairs and could also be associated with cognitive functioning.

In a large sample that combined 2 longitudinal population-based cohorts of twins, including 789 from Los Angeles and 2277 from Minnesota, Jackson and colleagues[82] examined change in 4 subtests of IQ from before cannabis initiation to the late teens. Of the four subtests, a measure assessing vocabulary knowledge showed an approximately 4-point decline in those who used cannabis during the follow-up period; unexpectedly, however, no relationship was found between cannabis frequency and IQ decline within the group of users. Furthermore, in a series of cotwin analyses, there was minimal evidence for greater IQ decline in twins who used cannabis (even frequently) compared with their nonusing twins. Similarly, in a longitudinal sample of 2232 British twins, Meier and colleagues[63] examined potential neuropsychological decline from age 12 to 18 by cannabis use. Adolescents who were dependent on cannabis at age 18 were found to have lower IQ at all timepoints (including before cannabis initiation), but cannabis dependence was not associated with IQ decline from age 12 to 18. Moreover, twins discordant for cannabis use showed minimal evidence of greater IQ decline or reductions in executive functioning compared with their cotwins. In a sample of 856 adolescent and young adult twins from Colorado, Ross and colleagues[83] used a cotwin design to examine associations between cannabis use, intelligence, and a well-validated battery of executive functioning measures. Overall, there was minimal evidence for associations between cannabis use and either intelligence or executive functioning after accounting for other substance use and within-family effects. In contrast to these studies, Ellingson and colleagues[84] recently found associations between cannabis use and memory using sibling-comparison analyses (not twins) that attempted to control for shared family effects. In a sample of 1192 adolescents drawn from substance abuse treatment programs, alternative schools, and juvenile probation departments in the US, cognitive functioning was assessed during adolescence (mean age 17.1–17.6) and young adulthood (mean age 23.5–23.8). In contrast to prior research, the authors reported minimal associations between cannabis use and cognitive functioning during adolescence. However, there were associations between the age of onset of regular cannabis use and verbal memory during young adulthood. Of note, there were no significant associations between cannabis use and measures of IQ or executive functioning at any timepoints.

There are 2 limitations to note regarding twin studies of cannabis use. First, despite the strength of this design to disentangle complex associations, most twin studies have had small numbers of frequent cannabis users and even fewer numbers of twins discordant for cannabis use. Second, no twin studies have examined these relationships over periods as long as Meier and colleagues,[78] and it is possible that cannabis-associated effects could emerge over longer periods.

Summary – Cannabis and Cognitive Functioning

Cross-sectional studies suggest cognitive reductions of a small magnitude in episodic memory, executive functioning, attention, and processing speed in adolescents who frequently use cannabis, especially in those who are treatment-seeking. However, abstinence from cannabis is associated with the attenuation of these reductions. Longitudinal studies are somewhat inconsistent but indicate that early and continued use of cannabis for longer periods of time (perhaps >10 years) may be associated with sustained cognitive decline, even with abstinence. Twin studies have challenged causal associations between cannabis and cognitive functioning in adolescence, suggesting that cognitive dysfunction might be associated with familial or shared environmental factors as opposed to cannabis-specific effects.

RESIDUAL EFFECTS – BRAIN STRUCTURE
Cross-Sectional Studies

Magnetic resonance imaging (MRI) studies in adolescents and young adults have examined differences between regular cannabis users and nonusers in several measures of brain structure, including volume of specific brain regions, thickness of the cerebral cortex, and density of brain gray matter. Early studies mostly used region of interest approaches to focus on brain regions with high densities of CB_1 receptors,[85] including subcortical structures such as the basal ganglia, hippocampus, and amygdala, as well as the cerebellum, cingulate cortex, and prefrontal cortex. However, consistent findings from initial studies in this area have been somewhat elusive, partially due to small sample sizes and variability in methodology.

Several cross-sectional studies found frequent cannabis use in adolescents and young adults was associated with smaller hippocampal volumes,[86-88] though other studies failed to replicate these differences.[89-92] Inconsistent results from cross-sectional studies were also reported in amygdala, striatum, cerebellum, orbitofrontal cortex, and cingulate cortex,[86,89,91,93-98] despite a high density of CB_1 receptors in these regions. Similarly, adolescent frequent cannabis users have been reported to have thinner prefrontal cortex compared with nonusers,[91,99] although several studies have not replicated these findings or have even found *thicker* prefrontal cortex in cannabis users.[90,100,101]

Larger cross-sectional studies have generally shown fewer consistent reductions in volume and cortical thickness in adolescent and young adult cannabis users. Weiland and colleagues[102] found no differences in measurements of subcortical volume, shape, or surface area in a sample of 50 adolescent daily cannabis users compared with nonusers. Similarly, in a sample of 439 adolescents, including 201 with weekly or greater cannabis frequency, Thayer and colleagues[103] found no associations between days of cannabis use in the prior 30 days and gray matter volumes, even when analyses were restricted to the sample of weekly users. In a sample of adolescents and young adults from the PNC, Scott and colleagues[104] found little evidence of dose–response relationships between cannabis use and brain volumes, cortical thickness, or gray matter density, and no age by group interactions suggesting adolescent vulnerability. One unique study examined links between cannabis use in adolescence, cortical thickness, and risk of schizophrenia by leveraging 3 large, population-based samples. French and colleagues[105] examined cortical thickness in 1574 participants between 12 and 21 years old and found a negative association between cannabis use by age 16 and cortical thickness, but only in men with a high polygenic risk score for schizophrenia (as determined by 108 genetic loci that had been identified at the time). The authors suggested that cortical thinning may mediate the link between cannabis use and risk of schizophrenia in men.

Two meta-analyses of cross-sectional structural neuroimaging studies in adolescent and young adult cannabis users have been conducted to date. A recent meta-analysis focused specifically on studies of cannabis users between 12 and 21 years old that used whole-brain voxel-based morphometry and voxelwise analyses to examine brain gray matter volume.[106] Unfortunately, this only included 6 total studies for meta-analysis. The authors reported that there were no significant differences between cannabis users and nonuser comparison groups when they synthesized results across studies. However, in follow-up meta-regressions, one region, the left superior temporal cortex, showed an increasing magnitude of differences between groups with age (ie, smaller volumes), suggesting a potential developmental gradient of cannabis associations. However, as the authors stated, as these results were not observed in primary analyses and were based on only 6 studies, they should be treated with caution. In a separate meta-analysis of volumetric structural neuroimaging findings associated with regular cannabis use, studies of adolescents and young adults comprised at least half of the 30 studies included.[8] Interestingly, findings synthesized from these cross-sectional studies suggested differences in hippocampal and orbitofrontal cortex volumes of a small magnitude in regular cannabis users, but minimal differences in other regions or in overall gray matter, white matter, or whole-brain volumes.

Longitudinal and Twin Studies

There have been few longitudinal studies of changes in brain structure associated with adolescent cannabis use or neuroimaging studies of twins discordant for cannabis use. However, such studies are crucial to increasing understanding of the potential impact of cannabis use on neurodevelopment, as shared familial factors may explain some brain structural differences seen in cannabis users[107] and some structural brain differences may predate and predict regular cannabis use. For example, several studies have shown that reduced volume of the orbitofrontal cortex is predictive of cannabis use during adolescence,[108–110] highlighting challenges in the interpretation of cross-sectional findings.

Longitudinal structural neuroimaging studies with small samples of adolescent cannabis users have shown conflicting findings. A study of 20 young adult heavy cannabis users found no structural differences in the hippocampus at either baseline or after approximately 3 years of cannabis use.[111] A 3-year longitudinal study of adolescent cannabis and alcohol users found reduced thinning of the cortex (ie, thicker cortex) in prefrontal, parietal, temporal, and occipital cortex, with greater cumulative marijuana use associated with increased thickness in temporal cortex at the follow-up visit.[101] Similarly, a small study of adolescent cannabis users followed over 18 months showed reduced levels of cortical thinning (ie, thicker cortex) in prefrontal, temporal, and parietal regions.[112] In contrast to findings of diminished cortical thickness from smaller studies, a recent, large-scale longitudinal study of 799 adolescents from the community-based IMAGEN cohort found that lifetime cannabis use was associated with *accelerated* cortical thinning from ages 14 to 19 in bilateral prefrontal cortex.[113] The regions that showed associations with cannabis use were also regions likely to show neurodevelopmental changes with age, providing some evidence for cannabis-associated changes in networks exhibiting protracted maturational trajectories.

Few studies have examined longer-term trajectories of brain structure in adolescent cannabis users. Using data from the Pittsburgh Youth Study, Meier and colleagues[114] used latent class growth analysis to identify different trajectories of adolescent cannabis use based on the annual assessments of cannabis use from ages 13 to 19 (n = 181). Despite identifying 4 trajectories of cannabis use during adolescence, they found no differences by a trajectory in cortical thickness, cortical volumes, or subcortical volumes when MRIs were acquired between ages 30 and 36.

To date, 2 cotwin studies have examined associations between cannabis use and brain structure in adolescence. In a sample of 436 young adult twins, Harper and colleagues[115] collected dimensional measures of cannabis use and alcohol use and examined their association with cortical thickness in specific networks of the brain that underlie functional systems of executive control and salience, including several regions in the prefrontal cortex. There were significant associations between alcohol abuse and reduced cortical thickness within these networks, and cotwin analyses indicated that these associations potentially reflected both familial factors and effects attributable to alcohol. However, there were no associations between cannabis and cortical thickness. Interestingly, in the same sample of twins, Harper and colleagues[116] found that alcohol use disorder and cannabis use disorder were both associated with reduced thickness of the medial (but not lateral) orbitofrontal cortex. Analyses of twins discordant for alcohol and cannabis use indicated that reductions in the medial orbitofrontal cortex seemed to be associated with both familial risk and substance effects.

Summary – Cannabis and Brain Structure

There is some initial evidence for alterations in the structure of the hippocampus and prefrontal cortex associated with cannabis use during adolescence, but significant heterogeneity exists in studies to date. Furthermore, some large-scale longitudinal research suggests that these structural brain changes are linked with cumulative cannabis use, but twin studies suggest that familial factors may contribute to brain changes associated with cannabis use. More prospective longitudinal studies and genetically informed designs are needed to assess the specific contribution of cannabis to structural brain alterations in adolescent cannabis users. Such studies are especially critical to disentangle substance-specific associations, as several different substances seem to share general associations with structural brain measures [117]

RESIDUAL EFFECTS – BRAIN FUNCTION

Several studies have examined potential differences in functional brain activation in adolescent frequent cannabis users using data collected during cognitive or emotional tasks (ie, task-based fMRI) or during rest (ie, resting-state fMRI). Several prior reviews have summarized these studies, and most have concluded that cannabis use during adolescence is associated with functional brain alterations [25,118–120] Yet, most findings are from small studies, and there is substantial inconsistency.

Early fMRI studies primarily used task-based approaches with small samples of adolescent cannabis users. Most studies found increased fMRI activation in "task positive" brain networks in adolescent cannabis users. For example, studies of working memory tasks have primarily reported increased prefrontal activation in adolescent cannabis users, despite showing equivalent task performance. [121–123] Similarly, 2 studies have reported increases in activation in prefrontal control networks associated with adolescent cannabis use during a task of response inhibition, [124,125] though another showed minimal group differences in fMRI during inhibition. [126] However, the interpretation of these data is not straightforward. To this end, studies of normative neurodevelopment have shown that "task positive" fMRI activation in the frontoparietal executive control network (FPN) during executive control tasks (eg, working memory and response inhibition) are associated with increasing age across development and improved task performance. [23,127] Thus, it is challenging to interpret increased activation in the FPN (whereby most of the reported activations would be localized) as reflecting abnormalities, as greater activation is consistently associated with better cognitive functioning in normative development. Larger studies with links between brain and behavior are needed to resolve this discrepancy.

There have also been fMRI studies of reward processing and emotion processing focusing on adolescent cannabis users. Studies of reward processing in adolescent cannabis users have not produced consistent findings to date. [128,129] However, a large study using an affective face processing task showed greater amygdala reactivity to angry faces in adolescent cannabis users, suggesting potential hypersensitivity to threat associated with cannabis. [130] Moreover, a follow-up study in the same cohort indicated that right amygdala hyperactivity to angry faces at baseline was a predictor of cannabis use (but not alcohol use) 5 years later, even in those who had not used cannabis at baseline. [131] These findings are intriguing and deserve replication and extension.

Two meta-analyses of the fMRI literature have been conducted to date but offer limited results. Blest-Hopley and colleagues [132] were only able to include 7 studies of adolescent cannabis users in a meta-analysis of whole-brain fMRI studies, finding significantly greater activation in adolescent cannabis users in the right inferior parietal gyrus and right putamen. In a separate meta-analysis, Blest-Hopley colleagues [133] only found 3 fMRI studies of adolescent cannabis users in which they acquired functional MRI data after 25 days of abstinence. Synthesizing results from these 3 studies suggested increased fMRI activation in abstinent adolescent cannabis users in regions of the dorsolateral and ventrolateral prefrontal and posterior parietal cortices, most of which are part of the FPN. However, as noted by the authors, all 3 articles were from the same laboratory and had some degree of overlapping samples, suggesting that the consistency of findings may be inflated.

Longitudinal and Twin Studies

In adolescent cannabis users, there have been no fMRI twin studies and only one longitudinal fMRI study. One small study (22 treatment-seeking adolescents with cannabis use disorder) reported decreased connectivity between caudal anterior cingulate cortex and dorsolateral and orbitofrontal cortices in adolescent cannabis users across 18 months.[134] Longitudinal changes in fMRI activation by cannabis use trajectories await further study.

Summary – Cannabis and Brain Function

There are relatively consistent findings from small studies of increased activation in "task positive" regions of the FPN in adolescent cannabis users, but the straightforward interpretation of these data is challenging. Unfortunately, fMRI research on adolescent cannabis use is subject to the same limitations as the cognitive and structural MRI research discussed above. As such, most fMRI studies in adolescent cannabis users have had small sample sizes, and many have included cannabis users with significant alcohol use, creating difficulties in the separation of risk factors. Some have not addressed issues of abstinence, which can impact measures of brain functioning.[123,135] As always, whether potential differences in fMRI measures are due to cannabis exposure is challenging to evaluate. For example, several studies have found that fMRI measures predict the initiation of cannabis use or problematic cannabis use during adolescence, including activation in regions of the FPN that overlap with those associated with cannabis use in cross-sectional studies.[37,136] Clearly, longitudinal research in larger samples is needed to replicate and expand on prior fMRI results.

SUMMARY

A substantial literature examining risks of adolescent cannabis use for brain and cognitive outcomes has amassed in the past 2 decades, but there is considerable heterogeneity in this research. Studies differ in the timeframe of measurements, frequency of use, measurements of cannabis quantity, types of cannabis used, and measures to assess neurocognitive functioning, brain structure, and brain functioning. This heterogeneity, combined with potential confounding and selection bias inherent in substance use research, has created challenges in interpreting this literature and reaching informed conclusions. However, at this point, several conclusions are warranted.

First, there is relatively consistent evidence that ongoing, frequent cannabis use is associated with small magnitude reductions in cognitive functioning. The clinical significance of these reductions is underexplored, as few studies have explored how such reductions are associated with functional outcomes.[61,78] However, an argument could be made that any reductions in cognitive functioning during continued periods of neurodevelopment are concerning from a public health standpoint. Moreover, even if adolescents eventually cease use, there is some evidence that frequent cannabis use during adolescence could reduce educational attainment[137] which could have downstream effects on occupational attainment and income.[138] Nonetheless, more research is needed to explore links between cannabis-associated cognitive deficits in adolescence and future educational, occupational, and psychosocial outcomes.

Second, there is relatively consistent evidence that abstinence is associated with improved cognitive functioning in cannabis users. The magnitude of this improvement is potentially dependent on the age at cannabis initiation and length of frequent cannabis use, although more research is needed to understand how these factors impact the recovery of function. In some cases, abstinence decreases the magnitude of reductions to levels that are indistinguishable from those of nonusers. However, achieving abstinence is challenging in individuals with cannabis dependence,[139] especially in individuals who establish patterns of frequent cannabis use in adolescence.[140] Thus, while it is potentially encouraging that abstinence may improve cognitive differences between cannabis users and nonusers, many adolescent-onset users are not able to achieve sustained abstinence.

Third, studies with longer follow-up periods (ie, >10 years) and with participants with the greatest cannabis frequency tend to show the strongest evidence of cannabis-related cognitive or IQ decline, while studies with shorter follow-up periods or lesser cannabis use tend to show limited associations after accounting for confounding factors, familial or genetic influences, and abstinence. This pattern is consistent with the hypothesis that cannabis-linked cognitive *impairments* after a period of abstinence are more likely to be evident after years of heavy cannabis use as opposed to shorter periods of regular use.[141]

Fourth, there are cognitive, brain structure, and brain activation differences (among other relevant factors) that seem to predict cannabis initiation/escalation or problematic substance use in general. These factors make straightforward interpretation of results challenging in this field. They also stress the need for multiple informative designs to triangulate evidence regarding the relationship between cannabis use in adolescence and brain-behavior functioning.

Finally, despite relevant mechanistic models and preclinical data, suggesting adolescent vulnerability to the brain effects of cannabis, there is mixed evidence for this vulnerability in humans to date. To this end, meta-analyses indicate that the magnitudes of neurocognitive effect sizes are remarkably similar in adult and adolescent frequent cannabis users. There are also limitations in research designs that attempt to examine heightened adolescent vulnerability to cannabis. Comparisons between early- and late-onset users are inconsistent in their definitions of early onset, and earlier age of onset is often associated with longer duration of use and heavier cannabis use,[61] creating challenges in isolating this effect. However, there is evidence from one rigorous longer-term longitudinal study of increased risk for poor cognitive functioning outcomes for those who initiate regular use in adolescence (compared with initiating use after age 18) and continue consistently using throughout adulthood.

Regardless of conclusions about cognitive and brain health, frequent cannabis use during adolescence is risky. This is especially true given the many unknowns left to discover with cannabis and the changing landscape of cannabis products available. There is also substantial variability in associations between cannabis and cognitive functioning; even with smaller effect sizes, frequent and prolonged cannabis use in adolescence may place certain vulnerable individuals at heightened risk of poor brain and behavior outcomes. Moreover, there are multiple pathways through which cannabis could influence health, and regular cannabis use during adolescence has been associated with several functionally relevant risks that are not discussed here, including increased likelihood of cannabis use disorder, increased risk for psychosis and schizophrenia, risks for poorer academic and occupational outcomes, and worsening of mental health conditions. These risks, in combination with potential risks for cognitive and brain functioning, highlight the potential benefits of delaying regular use of cannabis until early adulthood. Recommendations to adolescents from clinical providers and public health messengers should focus on such evidence-based assessments of risks.

Future Directions

While there has been substantial progress in studying cannabis use in adolescents over the past 2 decades, there are several areas of future research and development that are needed. There has been limited work to date regarding the chronic impact of different levels of THC or other cannabinoids on cognitive functioning, despite some data suggesting differential acute effects depending on cannabinoid constituents.[142,143] In addition, the literature on "synthetic cannabinoids" (eg, K2) is very limited at this time, and future work will need to examine how these substances may impact brain and cognitive functioning. There is also likely substantial variability in risk for brain-behavior problems associated with cannabis, and research into patient factors (eg, genomics) that may lead to adverse outcomes will be critical. Data from large-scale, population-representative studies will be essential to resolve many of the discrepancies described above and propel understanding of vulnerability in cannabis-associated brain-behavior effects. In the United States, the Adolescent Brain Cognitive Development study (https://abcdstudy.org) is acquiring repeated cognitive, mental health, and neuroimaging data on 10,000 adolescents starting from age 9 or 10, which will provide substantial data to answer critical questions about the risks of cannabis use in adolescence.

CLINICS CARE POINTS

- Frequent, active cannabis use in adolescents may be associated with small magnitude cognitive deficits in memory, attention, executive functioning, and speed of processing
- Adolescents who are frequent cannabis users are also likely to have psychiatric and substance use comorbidities that contribute to identified cognitive deficits
- Large magnitude cognitive deficits are less likely to be attributable to cannabis use
- Occasional cannabis use in adolescents is less likely to be associated with cognitive deficits except during the period in which an individual is intoxicated
- Abstinence from cannabis is likely to lead to some recovery in cognitive functioning
- Adolescent-onset, sustained, long-term use of cannabis may result in cognitive deficits that do not recover as readily with abstinence
- There are clear potential benefits of delaying regular use of cannabis until after the age of 18

FUNDING

Dr. Scott is supported by a United States (U.S.) Department of Veterans Affairs Merit Review Award (I01RX002699) and a grant from NIH (R01HD095278). The funders were not involved in the study design; collection, analysis, and interpretation of data; writing the report; or the decision to submit this article for publication.

REFERENCES

1. Substance Abuse and Mental Health Services Administration. Key substance use and mental health indicators in the United States: results from the 2020 national survey on drug use and health. Rockville, MD: Center for Behavioral

Health Statistics and Quality, Substance Abuse and Mental Health Services Administration; 2021. Available at: https://www.samhsa.gov/data/.

2. Miech RA, Johnston LD, O'Malley PM, et al. Monitoring the future national survey results on drug use, 1975-2020. Volume I, secondary school students. Ann Arbor, MI: Institute for Social Research, The University of Michigan; 2021. Available at: http://monitoringthefuture.org/pubs.html#monographs.

3. Miech RA, Patrick ME, O'Malley PM, et al. Trends in reported marijuana vaping among US adolescents, 2017-2019. JAMA 2020;323(5):475–6.

4. United Nations Office on Drugs and Crime. World drug report 2021. Vienna, Austria: United Nations Office on Drugs and Crime; 2021.

5. Volkow ND, Baler RD, Compton WM, et al. Adverse health effects of marijuana use. N Engl J Med 2014;370(23):2219–27.

6. Kendler KS, Schmitt E, Aggen SH, et al. Genetic and environmental influences on alcohol, caffeine, cannabis, and nicotine use from early adolescence to middle adulthood. Arch Gen Psychiatry 2008;65(6):674–82.

7. Ioannidis JPA. Why most published research findings are false. PLoS Med 2005; 2(8):e124.

8. Lorenzetti V, Chye Y, Silva P, et al. Does regular cannabis use affect neuroanatomy? An updated systematic review and meta-analysis of structural neuroimaging studies. Eur Arch Psychiatry Clin Neurosci 2019;269(1):59–71.

9. Scott JC, Slomiak ST, Jones JD, et al. Association of cannabis with cognitive functioning in adolescents and young adults: a systematic review and meta-analysis. JAMA Psychiatry 2018;75(6):585–95.

10. ElSohly M, Gul W. Constituents of cannabis sativa. In: Pertwee RG, editor. Handbook of cannabis. Oxford, UK: Oxford University Press; 2014. p. 3–22.

11. Grotenhermen F. Pharmacology of cannabinoids. Neuro Endocrinol Lett 2004; 25(1–2):14–23.

12. Mackie K. Distribution of cannabinoid receptors in the central and peripheral nervous system. Handbook Exp Pharmacol 2005;168:299–325.

13. Castillo PE, Younts TJ, Chávez AE, et al. Endocannabinoid signaling and synaptic function. Neuron 2012;76(1):70–81.

14. Harkany T, Guzmán M, Galve-Roperh I, et al. The emerging functions of endocannabinoid signaling during CNS development. Trends Pharmacol Sci 2007; 28(2):83–92.

15. Schneider M. Puberty as a highly vulnerable developmental period for the consequences of cannabis exposure. Addict Biol 2008;13(2):253–63.

16. Ellgren M, Artmann A, Tkalych O, et al. Dynamic changes of the endogenous cannabinoid and opioid mesocorticolimbic systems during adolescence: THC effects. Eur Neuropsychopharmacol 2008;18(11):826–34.

17. Meyer HC, Lee FS, Gee DG. The role of the endocannabinoid system and genetic variation in adolescent brain development. Neuropsychopharmacology 2018;43(1):21–33.

18. Galve-Roperh I, Palazuelos J, Aguado T, et al. The endocannabinoid system and the regulation of neural development: potential implications in psychiatric disorders. Eur Arch Psychiatry Clin Neurosci 2009;259(7):371–82.

19. Maccarone M, Guzmán M, Mackie K, et al. Programming of neural cells by (endo)cannabinoids: from physiological rules to emerging therapies. Nat Rev Neurosci 2014;15(12):786–801.

20. Gur RC, Richard J, Calkins ME, et al. Age group and sex differences in performance on a computerized neurocognitive battery in children age 8-21. Neuropsychology 2012;26(2):251–65.

21. Blakemore SJ, Choudhury S. Development of the adolescent brain: implications for executive function and social cognition. J Child Psychol Psychiatry 2006; 47(3–4):296–312.
22. Giedd JN, Blumenthal J, Jeffries NO, et al. Brain development during childhood and adolescence: a longitudinal MRI study. Nat Neurosci 1999;2(10):861–3.
23. Satterthwaite TD, Wolf DH, Erus G, et al. Functional maturation of the executive system during adolescence. J Neurosci 2013;33(41):16249–61.
24. Hadland SE, Knight JR, Harris SK. Medical marijuana: review of the science and implications for developmental-behavioral pediatric practice. J Dev Behav Pediatr 2015;36(2):115–23.
25. Jacobus J, Tapert SF. Effects of cannabis on the adolescent brain. Curr Pharm Des 2014;20(13):2186–93.
26. O'Shea M, Singh ME, McGregor IS, et al. Chronic cannabinoid exposure produces lasting memory impairment and increased anxiety in adolescent but not adult rats. J Psychopharmacol (Oxford) 2004;18(4):502–8.
27. Schneider M, Schömig E, Leweke FM. Acute and chronic cannabinoid treatment differentially affects recognition memory and social behavior in pubertal and adult rats. Addict Biol 2008;13(3–4):345–57.
28. Quinn HR, Matsumoto I, Callaghan PD, et al. Adolescent rats find repeated Delta(9)-THC less aversive than adult rats but display greater residual cognitive deficits and changes in hippocampal protein expression following exposure. Neuropsychopharmacology 2008;33(5):1113–26.
29. Rubino T, Realini N, Braida D, et al. Changes in hippocampal morphology and neuroplasticity induced by adolescent THC treatment are associated with cognitive impairment in adulthood. Hippocampus 2009;19(8):763–72.
30. Abush H, Akirav I. Short- and long-term cognitive effects of chronic cannabinoids administration in late-adolescence rats. PLoS One 2012;7(2):e31731.
31. Kirschmann EK, Pollock MW, Nagarajan V, et al. Effects of adolescent cannabinoid self-administration in rats on addiction-related behaviors and working memory. Neuropsychopharmacology 2017;42(5):989–1000.
32. Stinson FS, Ruan WJ, Pickering R, et al. Cannabis use disorders in the USA: prevalence, correlates and co-morbidity. Psychol Med 2006;36(10):1447–60.
33. Krueger RF, Hicks BM, Patrick CJ, et al. Etiologic connections among substance dependence, antisocial behavior, and personality: modeling the externalizing spectrum. J Abnorm Psychol 2002;111(3):411–24.
34. Jeffers AM, Glantz S, Byers A, et al. Sociodemographic Characteristics associated with and prevalence and frequency of cannabis use among adults in the US. JAMA Netw Open 2021;4(11):e2136571.
35. Duncan AE, Sartor CE, Scherrer JF, et al. The association between cannabis abuse and dependence and childhood physical and sexual abuse: evidence from an offspring of twins design. Addiction 2008;103(6):990–7.
36. Hasin DS, Kerridge BT, Saha TD, et al. Prevalence and correlates of DSM-5 cannabis use disorder, 2012-2013: findings from the national epidemiologic survey on alcohol and related Conditions-III. Am J Psychiatry 2016;173(6):588–99.
37. Spechler PA, Allgaier N, Chaarani B, et al. The initiation of cannabis use in adolescence is predicted by sex-specific psychosocial and neurobiological features. Eur J Neurosci 2019;50(3):2346–56.
38. Rohrer JM. Thinking clearly about correlations and Causation: graphical causal models for observational data. Adv Methods Practices Psychol Sci 2018;1(1):27–42.

39. Freeman TP, Lorenzetti V. Standard THC units": a proposal to standardize dose across all cannabis products and methods of administration. Addiction 2020; 115(7):1207–16.

40. Lorenzetti V, Hindocha C, Petrilli K, et al. The International Cannabis Toolkit (iCannToolkit): a multidisciplinary expert consensus on minimum standards for measuring cannabis use. Addiction 2021. https://doi.org/10.1111/add.15702.

41. Gelman A, Geurts HM. The statistical crisis in science: how is it relevant to clinical neuropsychology? Clin Neuropsychologist 2017;31(6–7):1000–14.

42. Munafò MR, Nosek BA, Bishop DVM, et al. A manifesto for reproducible science. Nat Hum Behav 2017;1:0021.

43. Botvinik-Nezer R, Holzmeister F, Camerer CF, et al. Variability in the analysis of a single neuroimaging dataset by many teams. Nature 2020;582(7810):84–8.

44. Poldrack RA, Baker CI, Durnez J, et al. Scanning the horizon: towards transparent and reproducible neuroimaging research. Nat Rev Neurosci 2017; 18(2):115–26.

45. Gelman A, Loken E. The garden of forking paths: why multiple comparisons can be a problem, even when there is no "fishing expedition" or "p-hacking" and the research hypothesis was posited ahead of time. New York, NY: Department of Statistics, Columbia University; 2013. p. 348.

46. Borgan F, Beck K, Butler E, et al. The effects of cannabinoid 1 receptor compounds on memory: a meta-analysis and systematic review across species. Psychopharmacology (Berl) 2019;236(11):3257–70.

47. Zhornitsky S, Pelletier J, Assaf R, et al. Acute effects of partial CB1 receptor agonists on cognition - a meta-analysis of human studies. Prog Neuropsychopharmacol Biol Psychiatry 2021;104:110063.

48. D'Souza DC, Ranganathan M, Braley G, et al. Blunted psychotomimetic and amnestic effects of delta-9-tetrahydrocannabinol in frequent users of cannabis. Neuropsychopharmacology 2008;33(10):2505–16.

49. Hart CL, Ilan AB, Gevins A, et al. Neurophysiological and cognitive effects of smoked marijuana in frequent users. Pharmacol Biochem Behav 2010;96(3): 333–41.

50. Dougherty DM, Mathias CW, Dawes MA, et al. Impulsivity, attention, memory, and decision-making among adolescent marijuana users. Psychopharmacology (Berl) 2013;226(2):307–19.

51. Harvey MA, Sellman JD, Porter RJ, et al. The relationship between non-acute adolescent cannabis use and cognition. Drug Alcohol Rev 2007;26(3):309–19.

52. Medina KL, Hanson KL, Schweinsburg AD, et al. Neuropsychological functioning in adolescent marijuana users: subtle deficits detectable after a month of abstinence. J Int Neuropsychol Soc 2007;13(5):807–20.

53. Solowij N, Jones KA, Rozman ME, et al. Verbal learning and memory in adolescent cannabis users, alcohol users and non-users. Psychopharmacology (Berl) 2011;216(1):131–44.

54. Ehrenreich H, Rinn T, Kunert HJ, et al. Specific attentional dysfunction in adults following early start of cannabis use. Psychopharmacology (Berl) 1999;142(3): 295–301.

55. Fontes MA, Bolla KI, Cunha PJ, et al. Cannabis use before age 15 and subsequent executive functioning. Br J Psychiatry 2011;198(6):442–7.

56. Gruber SA, Sagar KA, Dahlgren MK, et al. Age of onset of marijuana use and executive function. Psychol Addict Behav 2012;26(3):496–506.

57. Scott JC, Wolf DH, Calkins ME, et al. Cognitive functioning of adolescent and young adult cannabis users in the Philadelphia Neurodevelopmental Cohort. Psychol Addict Behav 2017;31(4):423–34.

58. Grant I, Gonzalez R, Carey CL, et al. Non-acute (residual) neurocognitive effects of cannabis use: a meta-analytic study. J Int Neuropsychol Soc 2003;9(5):679–89.

59. Schreiner AM, Dunn ME. Residual effects of cannabis use on neurocognitive performance after prolonged abstinence: a meta-analysis. Exp Clin Psychopharmacol 2012;20(5):420–9.

60. Bonnet U, Preuss UW. The cannabis withdrawal syndrome: current insights. Substance Abuse Rehabil 2017;2017(8):9–37.

61. Castellanos-Ryan N, Pingault JB, Parent S, et al. Adolescent cannabis use, change in neurocognitive function, and high-school graduation: a longitudinal study from early adolescence to young adulthood. Dev Psychopathol 2017;29(4):1253–66.

62. Infante MA, Nguyen-Louie TT, Worley M, et al. Neuropsychological trajectories associated with adolescent alcohol and cannabis use: a prospective 14-year study. J Int Neuropsychol Soc 2020;26(5):480–91.

63. Meier MH, Caspi A, Danese A, et al. Associations between adolescent cannabis use and neuropsychological decline: a longitudinal co-twin control study. Addiction 2018;113(2):257–65.

64. Morin JFG, Afzali MH, Bourque J, et al. A population-based analysis of the relationship between substance use and adolescent cognitive development. Am J Psychiatry 2019;176(2):98–106.

65. Giancola PR, Tarter RE. Executive cognitive functioning and risk for substance abuse. Psychol Sci 1999;10(3):203–5.

66. Sloboda Z, Glantz MD, Tarter RE. Revisiting the concepts of risk and protective factors for understanding the etiology and development of substance use and substance use disorders: implications for prevention. Subst Use Misuse 2012;47(8–9):944–62.

67. Tarter RE, Kirisci L, Mezzich A, et al. Neurobehavioral disinhibition in childhood predicts early age at onset of substance use disorder. Am J Psychiatry 2003;160(6):1078–85.

68. Becker MP, Collins PF, Schultz A, et al. Longitudinal changes in cognition in young adult cannabis users. J Clin Exp Neuropsychol 2018;40(6):529–43.

69. Hanson KL, Winward JL, Schweinsburg AD, et al. Longitudinal study of cognition among adolescent marijuana users over three weeks of abstinence. Addict Behav 2010;35(11):970–6.

70. Hanson KL, Thayer RE, Tapert SF. Adolescent marijuana users have elevated risk-taking on the balloon analog risk task. J Psychopharmacol (Oxford) 2014;28(11):1080–7.

71. Schuster RM, Gilman J, Schoenfeld D, et al. One Month of cannabis abstinence in adolescents and young adults is associated with improved memory. J Clin Psychiatry 2018;79(6):17m11977.

72. Wallace AL, Wade NE, Lisdahl KM. Impact of 2 Weeks of monitored abstinence on cognition in adolescent and young adult cannabis users. J Int Neuropsychol Soc 2020;26(8):776–84.

73. Fried PA, Watkinson B, Gray R. Neurocognitive consequences of marihuana–a comparison with pre-drug performance. Neurotoxicol Teratol 2005;27(2):231–9.

74. Hooper SR, Woolley D, De Bellis MD. Intellectual, neurocognitive, and academic achievement in abstinent adolescents with cannabis use disorder. Psychopharmacology (Berl) 2014;231(8):1467–77.

75. Pardini D, White HR, Xiong S, et al. Unfazed or dazed and confused: does early adolescent marijuana use cause sustained impairments in attention and academic functioning? J Abnorm Child Psychol 2015. https://doi.org/10.1007/s10802-015-0012-0.

76. Roten A, Baker NL, Gray KM. Cognitive performance in a placebo-controlled pharmacotherapy trial for youth with marijuana dependence. Addict Behav 2015;45:119–23.

77. Tait RJ, Mackinnon A, Christensen H. Cannabis use and cognitive function: 8-year trajectory in a young adult cohort. Addiction 2011;106(12):2195–203.

78. Meier MH, Caspi A, Ambler A, et al. Persistent cannabis users show neuropsychological decline from childhood to midlife. Proc Natl Acad Sci U S A 2012; 109(40):E2657–64.

79. Mokrysz C, Landy R, Gage SH, et al. Are IQ and educational outcomes in teenagers related to their cannabis use? A prospective cohort study. J Psychopharmacol 2016;30(2):159–68.

80. Mahedy L, Wootton R, Suddell S, et al. Testing the association between tobacco and cannabis use and cognitive functioning: findings from an observational and Mendelian randomization study. Drug Alcohol Depend 2021;221:108591.

81. Sanderson E, Glymour MM, Holmes MV, et al. Mendelian randomization. Nat Rev Methods Primers 2022;2(1):1–21.

82. Jackson NJ, Isen JD, Khoddam R, et al. Impact of adolescent marijuana use on intelligence: results from two longitudinal twin studies. Proc Natl Acad Sci U S A 2016;113(5):E500–8.

83. Ross JM, Ellingson JM, Rhee SH, et al. Investigating the causal effect of cannabis use on cognitive function with a quasi-experimental co-twin design. Drug Alcohol Depend 2020;206:107712.

84. Ellingson JM, Ross JM, Winiger E, et al. Familial factors may not explain the effect of moderate-to-heavy cannabis use on cognitive functioning in adolescents: a sibling-comparison study. Addiction 2021;116(4):833–44.

85. Glass M, Dragunow M, Faull RL. Cannabinoid receptors in the human brain: a detailed anatomical and quantitative autoradiographic study in the fetal, neonatal and adult human brain. Neuroscience 1997;77(2):299–318.

86. Ashtari M, Avants B, Cyckowski L, et al. Medial temporal structures and memory functions in adolescents with heavy cannabis use. J Psychiatr Res 2011;45(8): 1055–66.

87. Filbey FM, McQueeny T, Kadamangudi S, et al. Combined effects of marijuana and nicotine on memory performance and hippocampal volume. Behav Brain Res 2015;293:46–53.

88. Chye Y, Suo C, Yücel M, et al. Cannabis-related hippocampal volumetric abnormalities specific to subregions in dependent users. Psychopharmacology (Berl) 2017;234(14):2149–57.

89. Cousijn J, Wiers RW, Ridderinkhof KR, et al. Grey matter alterations associated with cannabis use: results of a VBM study in heavy cannabis users and healthy controls. Neuroimage 2012;59(4):3845–51.

90. Kumra S, Robinson P, Tambyraja R, et al. Parietal lobe volume deficits in adolescents with schizophrenia and adolescents with cannabis use disorders. J Am Acad Child Adolesc Psychiatry 2012;51(2):171–80.

91. Mashhoon Y, Sava S, Sneider JT, et al. Cortical thinness and volume differences associated with marijuana abuse in emerging adults. Drug Alcohol Depend 2015;155:275–83.
92. Medina KL, McQueeny T, Nagel BJ, et al. Prefrontal cortex morphometry in abstinent adolescent marijuana users: subtle gender effects. Addict Biol 2009;14(4):457–68.
93. Battistella G, Fornari E, Annoni JM, et al. Long-term effects of cannabis on brain structure. Neuropsychopharmacology 2014;39(9):2041–8.
94. Block RI, O'Leary DS, Ehrhardt JC, et al. Effects of frequent marijuana use on brain tissue volume and composition. Neuroreport 2000;11(3):491–6.
95. Churchwell JC, Lopez-Larson M, Yurgelun-Todd DA. Altered frontal cortical volume and decision making in adolescent cannabis users. Front Psychol 2010; 1:225.
96. Cohen M, Rasser PE, Peck G, et al. Cerebellar grey-matter deficits, cannabis use and first-episode schizophrenia in adolescents and young adults. Int J Neuropsychopharmacol 2012;15(3):297–307.
97. Medina KL, Nagel BJ, Tapert SF. Abnormal cerebellar morphometry in abstinent adolescent marijuana users. Psychiatry Res 2010;182(2):152–9.
98. Price JS, McQueeny T, Shollenbarger S, et al. Effects of marijuana use on prefrontal and parietal volumes and cognition in emerging adults. Psychopharmacology (Berl) 2015;232(16):2939–50.
99. Lopez-Larson MP, Bogorodzki P, Rogowska J, et al. Altered prefrontal and insular cortical thickness in adolescent marijuana users. Behav Brain Res 2011;220(1):164–72.
100. Filbey FM, McQueeny T, DeWitt SJ, et al. Preliminary findings demonstrating latent effects of early adolescent marijuana use onset on cortical architecture. Dev Cogn Neurosci 2015;16:16–22.
101. Jacobus J, Squeglia LM, Meruelo AD, et al. Cortical thickness in adolescent marijuana and alcohol users: a three-year prospective study from adolescence to young adulthood. Dev Cogn Neurosci 2015;16:101–9.
102. Weiland BJ, Thayer RE, Depue BE, et al. Daily marijuana use is not associated with brain morphometric measures in adolescents or adults. J Neurosci 2015; 35(4):1505–12.
103. Thayer RE, YorkWilliams S, Karoly HC, et al. Structural neuroimaging correlates of alcohol and cannabis use in adolescents and adults. Addiction 2017;112(12): 2144–54.
104. Scott JC, Rosen AFG, Moore TM, et al. Cannabis use in youth is associated with limited alterations in brain structure. Neuropsychopharmacology 2019;44(8): 1362–9.
105. French L, Gray C, Leonard G, et al. Early cannabis use, polygenic risk score for schizophrenia and brain maturation in adolescence. JAMA Psychiatry 2015; 72(10):1002–11.
106. Allick A, Park G, Kim K, et al. Age- and sex-related cortical gray matter volume differences in adolescent cannabis users: a systematic review and meta-analysis of voxel-based morphometry studies. Front Psychiatry 2021;12:745193.
107. Pagliaccio D, Barch DM, Bogdan R, et al. Shared predisposition in the association between cannabis use and subcortical brain structure. JAMA Psychiatry 2015;72(10):994–1001.
108. Cheetham A, Allen NB, Whittle S, et al. Orbitofrontal volumes in early adolescence predict initiation of cannabis use: a 4-year longitudinal and prospective study. Biol Psychiatry 2012;71(8):684–92.

109. Luby JL, Agrawal A, Belden A, et al. Developmental trajectories of the orbito-frontal cortex and anhedonia in middle childhood and risk for substance use in adolescence in a longitudinal sample of depressed and healthy preschoolers. Am J Psychiatry 2018;175(10):1010–21.
110. Wade NE, Bagot KS, Cota CI, et al. Orbitofrontal cortex volume prospectively predicts cannabis and other substance use onset in adolescents. J Psychopharmacol 2019;33(9):1124–31.
111. Koenders L, Lorenzetti V, de Haan L, et al. Longitudinal study of hippocampal volumes in heavy cannabis users. J Psychopharmacol 2017;31(8):1027–34.
112. Epstein KA, Kumra S. Altered cortical maturation in adolescent cannabis users with and without schizophrenia. Schizophr Res 2015;162(1–3):143–52.
113. Albaugh MD, Ottino-Gonzalez J, Sidwell A, et al. Association of cannabis use during adolescence with neurodevelopment. JAMA Psychiatry 2021;78(9):1–11.
114. Meier MH, Schriber RA, Beardslee J, et al. Associations between adolescent cannabis use frequency and adult brain structure: a prospective study of boys followed to adulthood. Drug Alcohol Depend 2019;202:191–9.
115. Harper J, Malone SM, Wilson S, et al. The effects of alcohol and cannabis use on the cortical thickness of cognitive control and salience brain networks in emerging adulthood: a Co-twin control study. Biol Psychiatry 2021;89(10):1012–22.
116. Harper J, Wilson S, Malone SM, et al. Orbitofrontal cortex thickness and sub-stance use disorders in emerging adulthood: causal inferences from a co-twin control/discordant twin study. Addiction 2021;116(9):2548–58.
117. Mackey S, Allgaier N, Chaarani B, et al. Mega-analysis of gray matter volume in substance dependence: general and substance-specific regional effects. Am J Psychiatry 2019;176(2):119–28.
118. Blest-Hopley G, Colizzi M, Giampietro V, et al. Is the adolescent brain at greater vulnerability to the effects of cannabis? A narrative review of the evidence. Front Psychiatry 2020;11:859.
119. Lees B, Debenham J, Squeglia LM. Alcohol and cannabis use and the devel-oping brain. Alcohol Res 2021;41(1):11.
120. Lisdahl KM, Gilbart ER, Wright NE, et al. Dare to delay? The impacts of adoles-cent alcohol and marijuana use onset on cognition, brain structure, and function. Front Psychiatry 2013;4:53.
121. Jager G, Block RI, Luijten M, et al. Cannabis use and memory brain function in adolescent boys: a cross-sectional multicenter functional magnetic resonance im-aging study. J Am Acad Child Adolesc Psychiatry 2010;49(6):561–72, 572.e1-3.
122. Schweinsburg AD, Nagel BJ, Schweinsburg BC, et al. Abstinent adolescent marijuana users show altered fMRI response during spatial working memory. Psychiatry Res 2008;163(1):40–51.
123. Schweinsburg AD, Schweinsburg BC, Medina KL, et al. The influence of recency of use on fMRI response during spatial working memory in adolescent marijuana users. J Psychoactive Drugs 2010;42(3):401–12.
124. Tapert SF, Schweinsburg AD, Drummond SPA, et al. Functional MRI of inhibitory processing in abstinent adolescent marijuana users. Psychopharmacology (Berl) 2007;194(2):173–83.
125. Wallace AL, Maple KE, Barr AT, et al. BOLD responses to inhibition in cannabis-using adolescents and emerging adults after 2 weeks of monitored cannabis abstinence. Psychopharmacology (Berl) 2020;237(11):3259–68.
126. Behan B, Connolly CG, Datwani S, et al. Response inhibition and elevated parietal-cerebellar correlations in chronic adolescent cannabis users. Neuro-pharmacology 2014;84:131–7.

127. Zuo N, Salami A, Yang Y, et al. Activation-based association profiles differentiate network roles across cognitive loads. Hum Brain Mapp 2019;40(9):2800–12.
128. Jager G, Block RI, Luijten M, et al. Tentative evidence for striatal hyperactivity in adolescent cannabis-using boys: a cross-sectional multicenter fMRI study. J Psychoactive Drugs 2013;45(2):156–67.
129. Karoly HC, Bryan AD, Weiland BJ, et al. Does incentive-elicited nucleus accumbens activation differ by substance of abuse? An examination with adolescents. Dev Cogn Neurosci 2015;16:5–15.
130. Spechler PA, Orr CA, Chaarani B, et al. Cannabis use in early adolescence: evidence of amygdala hypersensitivity to signals of threat. Dev Cogn Neurosci 2015;16:63–70.
131. Spechler PA, Chaarani B, Orr C, et al. Longitudinal associations between amygdala reactivity and cannabis use in a large sample of adolescents. Psychopharmacology (Berl) 2020;237(11):3447–58.
132. Blest-Hopley G, Giampietro V, Bhattacharyya S. Residual effects of cannabis use in adolescent and adult brains - a meta-analysis of fMRI studies. Neurosci Biobehav Rev 2018;88:26–41.
133. Blest-Hopley G, Giampietro V, Bhattacharyya S. Regular cannabis use is associated with altered activation of central executive and default mode networks even after prolonged abstinence in adolescent users: results from a complementary meta-analysis. Neurosci Biobehav Rev 2019;96:45–55.
134. Camchong J, Lim KO, Kumra S. Adverse effects of cannabis on adolescent brain development: a longitudinal study. Cereb Cortex 2017;27(3):1922–30.
135. Jacobus J, Goldenberg D, Wierenga CE, et al. Altered cerebral blood flow and neurocognitive correlates in adolescent cannabis users. Psychopharmacology (Berl) 2012;222(4):675–84.
136. Tervo-Clemmens B, Simmonds D, Calabro FJ, et al. Early cannabis use and neurocognitive risk: a prospective functional neuroimaging study. Biol Psychiatry Cogn Neurosci Neuroimaging 2018;3(8):713–25.
137. Schaefer JD, Hamdi NR, Malone SM, et al. Associations between adolescent cannabis use and young-adult functioning in three longitudinal twin studies. Proc Natl Acad Sci U S A 2021;118(14). e2013180118.
138. Danielsson AK, Falkstedt D, Hemmingsson T, et al. Cannabis use among Swedish men in adolescence and the risk of adverse life course outcomes: results from a 20 year-follow-up study. Addiction 2015;110(11):1794–802.
139. Budney AJ, Sofis MJ, Borodovsky JT. An update on cannabis use disorder with comment on the impact of policy related to therapeutic and recreational cannabis use. Eur Arch Psychiatry Clin Neurosci 2019;269(1):73–86.
140. Zehra A, Burns J, Liu CK, et al. Cannabis addiction and the brain: a review. J Neuroimmune Pharmacol 2018;13(4):438–52.
141. National Academies of Sciences, Engineering, and Medicine. The health effects of cannabis and cannabinoids: the current state of evidence and recommendations for research. Washington, DC: The National Academies Press; 2017.
142. Morgan CJA, Schafer G, Freeman TP, et al. Impact of cannabidiol on the acute memory and psychotomimetic effects of smoked cannabis: naturalistic study. Br J Psychiatry 2010;197(4):285–90.
143. Rømer Thomsen K, Callesen MB, Feldstein Ewing SW. Recommendation to reconsider examining cannabis subtypes together due to opposing effects on brain, cognition and behavior. Neurosci Biobehav Rev 2017;80:156–8.

The Effects of Adolescent Cannabis Use on Psychosocial Functioning
A Critical Review of the Evidence

Jonathan D. Schaefer, PhD, Kayla M. Nelson, BS, Sylia Wilson, PhD*

KEYWORDS

- Cannabis • Psychosocial functioning • Interpersonal relationships • Education
- Socioeconomic status

KEY POINTS

- Observational studies have shown that cannabis use in adolescence is consistently associated with impairments in multiple domains of psychosocial functioning, including interpersonal relationships, academics, and socioeconomic attainment. Cannabis use is also associated with increased risk of legal consequences.
- The mechanisms responsible for these associations are largely unclear. Although it is reasonable to assume that associations reflect a causal effect of cannabis on functioning, it is also possible that they arise due to reverse causation or confounding by shared vulnerability factors.
- Causally informative studies are key to differentiating between these possibilities. However, these designs have focused primarily on educational and socioeconomic outcomes to date, leaving the causal status of associations between cannabis use and other important psychosocial outcomes uncertain.

INTRODUCTION

Cannabis use in adolescence has been consistently linked to a range of negative psychosocial outcomes, including problematic peer, romantic, and parent–child relationships, worse educational outcomes, lower adult socioeconomic status, and legal consequences. In this narrative review, we present key findings from research published in the past 20 years on long-term psychosocial outcomes in adolescents who

This article originally appeared in *Child and Adolescent Psychiatric Clinics*, Volume 32 Issue 1, January 2023.

Institute of Child Development, University of Minnesota, 51 East River Parkway, Minneapolis, MN 55455, USA

* Corresponding author.

E-mail address: syliaw@umn.edu

Twitter: @JonSchaeferPhD (J.D.S.); @KaylaNelson (K.M.N.); @WilsonSylia (S.W.)

use cannabis. We first summarize current evidence from relevant longitudinal studies. Because we focus on long-term psychosocial outcomes, findings from these studies may reflect cumulative effects of adolescent cannabis use, as well as those of repeated cannabis exposure into adulthood—although in some cases, long-term outcomes (eg, justice system involvement) may be driven simply by possession of cannabis, the shorter-term consequences of use, or acute intoxication. We use the term "cannabis use" broadly to encompass the varying definitions in these studies, providing more precise descriptors (ie, in terms of cannabis use disorder status or cannabis use frequency) when possible. We then consider evidence for potential mechanisms linking adolescent cannabis use and long-term psychosocial outcomes, drawing largely from the smaller number of relevant causally informative studies, which include those conducting sibling/twin comparisons or taking advantage of "natural experiments" (eg, changes in the legal status of cannabis). We critically consider the current evidence base for concluding the causal effects of adolescent cannabis use on psychosocial functioning, given methodological and study design limitations. Finally, we offer suggestions for future investigations seeking to identify causal mechanisms and clinic care points for clinical providers and public policy makers concerned with adolescent cannabis use and its effects on later psychosocial outcomes.

Current Evidence

There is extensive evidence from research published over the past 20 years that adolescent cannabis use is associated with negative outcomes in important psychosocial domains, including functioning in peer and romantic relationships, the quality of the parent-child relationship, educational outcomes, adult socioeconomic status, and legal consequences (**Box 1**).

Peer and romantic relationships

Decades of research on substance use have sought to understand its associations with functioning in peer and romantic relationships, given the importance of these social bonds for well-being.[1,2] Cannabis use is associated with decreased social network size and, in turn, lower perceived social support.[3] A number of studies

---

Box 1
Psychosocial outcomes

Interpersonal relationships
- Social network size and support
- Relationship quality/satisfaction
- Attachment
- Delinquent/substance-using peers
- Sexual behavior
- Parental monitoring/knowledge

Socioeconomic status
- School performance and drop-out
- Educational attainment
- Employment and occupational prestige
- Income and debt

Legal
- Driving while intoxicated
- Car crashes
- Delinquency
- Justice system involvement

have examined the role of peers in adolescent cannabis use, inferring a causal pathway from peer relationships to cannabis initiation and use in adolescence.[4–6] However, there is some evidence that the direction of the effect may be reversed, so that early-onset cannabis use, in adolescence, leads to later associations with delinquent and substance-using peers.[7,8] Regular cannabis use in adolescence and early adulthood has also been found to be associated with lower likelihood of being in a romantic relationship.[9] For those who are in romantic relationships, adolescent cannabis use is associated with lower levels of relationship satisfaction, even after accounting for other potential confounders, such as comorbid substance use, family functioning, and psychopathology.[10] There is also evidence of greater engagement in risky sexual behaviors among women who first initiated cannabis use in adolescence relative to those who first initiated in early adulthood or later.[11] Taken together, evidence from these longitudinal studies suggests that adolescent cannabis use is associated with smaller social networks, lower social support, fewer peer and romantic relationships, greater affiliation with deviant and substance-using peers, lower romantic relationship satisfaction, and more risky sexual behaviors.

Parent–child relationships
Parent–child relationships continue to serve as a key source of support and guidance for adolescents as they become increasingly independent in later adolescence and early adulthood.[12] Most studies examining associations between these relationships and cannabis use have examined how different aspects of the parent–child relationship and specific parenting behaviors relate to cannabis initiation and course of use in adolescence. Collectively, these studies suggest that the quality of the parent–child relationship, parental monitoring, household rules about cannabis and other substance use, and parents' knowledge of their adolescents, their peers, and their activities may act as particularly important buffers against cannabis initiation, use, and negative consequences of use.[13,14] There is also evidence that parental factors can moderate the negative influences of deviant peers on adolescent cannabis use.[15] Fewer studies have considered potential effects of adolescent cannabis use on parent–child relationship quality. Qualitative studies suggest adolescent cannabis use is associated with more problematic interactions and relationships with family members.[16,17] Similarly, research seeking to understand the bidirectional nature of adolescent cannabis use and family relationships has shown that externalizing behavior in early adolescence, which has been linked to substance use, is negatively associated with the quality of the parent–child relationship.[18] One meta-analysis found that the association between earlier relationship experiences and later substance use was significantly stronger than that between earlier substance use and later attachment in adulthood.[19] This suggests that, perhaps, parent–child relationships may affect later substance use more than substance use affects parent–child relationships. However, even longitudinal studies of this kind are not sufficient to determine a causal pathway in either direction. Taken together, evidence from the existing longitudinal studies considering adolescent cannabis use and functioning in the parent–child relationship suggests that lower parental monitoring and knowledge are associated with adolescent cannabis use, and that adolescent cannabis use may be associated with lower-quality parent–child relationships.

School performance and educational attainment
An extensive body of longitudinal studies has considered associations between adolescent cannabis use and school performance and educational attainment. Several systematic reviews conducted over the past several decades find that

adolescent cannabis use is associated with increased risk of school drop-out and lower educational attainment.[20–22] However, as these reviews note, many (though not all) of the existing studies find that associations between adolescent cannabis use and educational outcomes are dramatically attenuated after accounting for potential confounders, including family demographics, child cognitive ability at baseline, and behavior problems.[21,23]

Adult socioeconomic status

A substantial body of research has considered associations between cannabis use in adulthood and financial and job-related outcomes. In contrast, there are markedly fewer longitudinal studies considering longer-term associations between adolescent cannabis use and adult socioeconomic outcomes. Still, the existing studies paint a relatively consistent picture, indicating that greater cannabis use or more chronic patterns of use in adolescence are associated with greater risk of unemployment, lower occupational prestige, lower income, greater debt, and more difficulty paying for medical necessities in young or middle adulthood.[24–26] These findings are largely mirrored by longitudinal studies in adulthood, which indicate that greater cannabis use at baseline is prospectively associated with greater risk of unemployment, lower income, and job loss among people used at baseline.[27–30] Notably, although findings from these longitudinal studies are remarkably consistent in suggesting that both adolescent and adult cannabis use are associated with varied indicators of adult socioeconomic status, many of these studies also indicate that associations between cannabis use and adult socioeconomic outcomes are significantly moderated by several factors, including income, race/ethnicity, sex, and age of cannabis initiation. For example, associations between cannabis use and risk of job loss were found to be are highest at the lowest and highest extremes of the income distribution, though the mechanisms driving this finding are as yet unclear.[29] Adolescent cannabis use was also prospectively associated with lower occupational prestige and lower income among White participants, but not Black participants, in a United States sample.[31] Another study of a nationally representative sample of United States high school seniors (from the classes of 1976–1988) reported that frequent cannabis use was prospectively associated with lower occupational attainment 10 years later among men, but not among women.[32] Finally, a study of the 2015 National Survey of Drug Use and Health (NSDUH) found that adolescents who initiated cannabis use earlier had lower odds of graduating from high school and greater risk of unemployment relative to those who initiated cannabis later.[33] Taken together, however, the literature on adolescent and adult cannabis use paint a relatively consistent picture, indicating that greater use is associated with unemployment, lower occupational prestige, lower income, job loss, and greater debt in adulthood.

Legal consequences

There is considerable interest in the potential legal consequences of adolescent cannabis use. Most of the research in this area has focused on cross-sectional associations between cannabis use in adolescence and risky behavior (eg, driving while intoxicated, car crashes), delinquency, and justice system involvement, with markedly fewer longitudinal studies considering longer-term associations with legal consequences in adulthood. Adolescent cannabis use, and particularly early cannabis initiation, has been found to be associated with greater criminal involvement and delinquency in later adolescence and adulthood.[7,34,35] However, the direction of this association remains unclear, and there is evidence that adolescents higher in behavioral disinhibition and risk proneness are also more likely to initiate cannabis use and use more cannabis.[36,37] Of note, one rationale for more permissive cannabis laws (medical and recreational cannabis legalization) is to reduce racial/ethnic inequities in law enforcement and inequities in legal consequences for cannabis use (eg, disproportionate number of arrests for cannabis use and possession of people who are Black, though rates of use are similar among people who are Black and White).[38] Taken together, evidence from the relatively small number of longitudinal studies considering adolescent cannabis use and legal consequences suggests that adolescent cannabis use is associated with risky behavior, delinquency, and justice system involvement in adolescence and adulthood, though it remains unclear whether this reflects causal effects.

CONSIDERATIONS

Although links between adolescent cannabis use and psychosocial impairment in both adolescence and adulthood are well established, the mechanisms underlying these links remain largely unclear. Unfortunately, methodological limitations have seriously limited the inferences and conclusions that can be drawn regarding the mechanistic links between adolescent cannabis use and long-term psychosocial functioning outcomes in adulthood.

Limitations of Current Evidence

Methodological limitations to studies of adolescent cannabis use and psychosocial functioning outcomes include issues of sample ascertainment, measurement, and study design, which result in limited generalizability of findings to the broader population and serious risk of study confounding (**Box 2**). Sample ascertainment bias resulting from inadequate identification or enrollment of a representative sample and differential attrition due to factors relevant to cannabis use or psychosocial impairment, or both, have the potential to limit the generalizability of findings and substantially bias results. Measurement issues include unreliability of measurement, overreliance on the use of retrospective self-reports to assess cannabis use, and the difficulty of establishing a standard cannabis "dose" in a way similar to the measurement of alcohol (eg, a standard drink) or nicotine (eg, a cigarette), given different routes of cannabis administration and variation in THC concentrations across cannabis products. Studies also commonly use different definitions of "use," ranging from quantity or frequency of cannabis use to a diagnosis of cannabis use disorder. Perhaps the most serious methodological limitation is that most study designs cannot

---

Box 2
Methodological limitations

Sample ascertainment
• Nonrepresentative samples
• Differential attrition

Measurement
• Unreliability
• Retrospective self-reports
• Nonstandard cannabis "dose"
• Nonstandard definitions of cannabis "use"

Study designs
• Correlational/observational
• Unaccounted confounding factors

adequately account for confounding factors. Many studies have attempted to "control" or statistically account for putative confounders, including demographic characteristics and socioeconomic factors (eg, sex, race/ethnicity, socioeconomic status), as well as other potentially important moderators (eg, parental substance use disorder, age of cannabis initiation, cohort effects such as cannabis legalization). However, attempts to statistically account for confounders by including additional variables in statistical models are necessarily limited to those putative confounders/moderators identified and measured by researchers, which may or may not adequately reflect or capture the entire universe of confounders, and are themselves subject to measurement issues, including unreliability in measurement and reliance on retrospective self-reports that may be distorted by well-known cognitive biases.[39]

Alternative Mechanistic Explanations for Adolescent Cannabis Use and Psychosocial Functioning Links

The predominant explanation for links between adolescent cannabis use and psychosocial functioning outcomes posits causal effects of cannabis on brain integrity,[40,41] which results in poorer cognitive performance and difficulties with emotion regulation[20,42] or amotivation[43] and consequent impairment in important domains of psychosocial functioning. This explanation is consistent with findings from the experimental animal literature, which clearly indicates that heavy, chronic substance use causally and adversely affects the brain, including during the critical adolescent period of rapid brain development.[44] However, in experimental animal studies, it is possible to randomly assign animals to the administration of a defined quantity of cannabis exposure, thereby isolating the putative causal mechanism. This is simply not possible in human studies—it is not ethical to randomly assign adolescents to cannabis exposure. This means that any preexisting factors that might lead some adolescents to initiate cannabis use or to use more cannabis than other adolescents may confound study results, and it is not possible to isolate cannabis exposure, as opposed to these other confounding factors, as the causal factor for psychosocial impairment. That is, associations between adolescent cannabis use and negative psychosocial outcomes may be due primarily (or entirely) to confounding by shared vulnerability factors that account for both initiation and use of cannabis in adolescence and concurrent and subsequent psychosocial impairment. This alternative explanation warrants serious consideration, given converging streams of evidence suggesting that many forms of psychosocial adversity (eg, maltreatment or socioeconomic disadvantage) occur disproportionately among individuals who use cannabis.[45,46]

Evidence from Causally Informative Studies

Fortunately, there are study designs that allow us to approximate an experiment, even when true random assignment is not possible—natural experiments or quasi-experimental study designs[47,48] (**Box 3**). Although these quasi-experimental approaches cannot yield findings that are as definitive as a true experiment, when multiple such study designs are used in a complementary manner and yield converging findings, our confidence in causal inferences is considerably increased. Relevant study designs include discordant sibling designs (and the even more informative variant, discordant twin designs), Mendelian randomization studies, and quasi-interventions, such as changes in the legal status of cannabis or age of legal use. Unfortunately, to our knowledge, these more causally informative approaches have so far been almost exclusively limited to the examination of educational outcomes and adult socioeconomic indicators, meaning evidence for a specific causal pathway for the effects of cannabis use in adolescence on functioning in peer, romantic, or parent–child

Box 3
Causally informative study designs

Approach	Definition	Strengths	Limitations
Discordant sibling/twin design	Compares outcomes when (twin) siblings are discordant in their cannabis use. If the effects of cannabis are causal, then the sibling reporting more cannabis use should experience the outcome at higher levels than their less-cannabis-using sibling.	Controls for confounding by shared genetics and environment.	Potential for confounding by factors NOT perfectly shared by siblings; affected more strongly by measurement error; limited power.
Mendelian randomization (MR)	MR uses one or more genetic variants associated with cannabis use as an instrumental variable to test the causal effect of cannabis use on an outcome.	Genetic variants are not subject to confounding from environmental factors and cannot be caused by the outcome, so this approach controls for confounding by shared genetics and environment, reverse causality, and selection bias. Genetic variants also do not change over time and are measured with high accuracy, reducing measurement error.	Generally low power, possibility of biased estimates due to horizontal pleiotropy, population stratification, assortative mating, or dynastic effects.
Quasi-interventions	Capitalizes on an external event or intervention occurring at a specific timepoint that affects cannabis use in one population but not another in a quasi-random fashion (eg, changes in cannabis legalization). These populations are then compared with see if the population with greater cannabis exposure or access experiences a higher proportion of negative outcomes.	Can include study settings that would be impractical or unethical to produce by researchers; addresses confounding by genetics and environment and reverse causality.	Possibility of selection bias if "exposed" and "unexposed" groups are not sufficiently comparable (ie, some unobserved confounding may remain).

relationship domains, or legal consequences, is seriously limited (see[49,50]; but see also[51]). Nonetheless, although small in number, the relevant causally informative studies of adolescent cannabis use and educational and socioeconomic outcomes are informative. One study among adult male twins who served in the US military during the Vietnam era found that twin differences in retrospectively reported adolescent cannabis use and cannabis dependence in adolescence were not associated with educational attainment.[52] A second study of a community-based sample of adult Australian twins found that although retrospectively-reported adolescent cannabis use was associated with risk of school dropout, this association was not observed at the within-pair level (ie, even among twin pairs differing in their levels of cannabis use, both twins were at increased risk of school dropout), suggesting shared vulnerability factors account for the association, rather than a causal effect of cannabis exposure.[53] In contrast to these earlier studies, a more recent, prospective study of 3 community-based samples of Minnesota same-sex twins found among monozygotic twin pairs differing in their levels of cannabis use, the twin who used more cannabis in adolescence also had lower educational attainment, occupational prestige, and income in young adulthood than their lesser-using cotwin, consistent with a potential causal effect of cannabis exposure on adult socioeconomic outcomes.[54] It is possible that these discrepant findings arise due to differences in statistical power, as the Schaefer and colleagues (2021) study is the only causally informative analysis we are aware of that used continuous measures of both cannabis use and educational outcomes (rather than dichotomous indicators such as early vs cannabis later use, or high school graduation vs school dropout). Another study took advantage of a change in the regulation of cannabis sales in Dutch coffee shops to assess the effects of cannabis use on university students' school performance.[55] To reduce drug tourism, the city of Maastricht in the Netherlands enacted restrictions on the nationality of students who could purchase cannabis in coffee shops in the city—students from the Netherlands, Belgium, and Germany could access coffee shops while students from France and Luxembourg could not. Among the students who could no longer legally buy cannabis in coffee shops, grades improved by 0.10 of a standard deviation relative to the students who could still buy cannabis, and their course pass rates improved by 5%, with gains that were 3.5 times greater in courses that required numerical/mathematical skills. These findings are consistent with a causal effect of cannabis exposure on educational outcomes, though an important limitation is that, because many students were likely able to acquire cannabis from other students still able to buy cannabis, it is possible the study underestimated the effects of a true ban. Taken together, evidence from the as yet relatively small number of causally informative studies considering adolescent cannabis and psychosocial outcomes suggests that adolescent cannabis use may be causally associated with poorer school performance, lower educational attainment, lower occupational prestige, and lower income in adulthood, even accounting for other shared vulnerability factors.

SUMMARY

Adolescent cannabis use is associated with negative outcomes in a range of important psychosocial domains. Although the existing literature varies somewhat by psychosocial domain, there is consistent evidence that adolescent cannabis use is associated with impairment in peer, romantic, and parent–child relationship domains; poorer school performance and lower educational attainment; lower adult socioeconomic status; and legal consequences. Although these associations are often considered to reflect a causal effect of cannabis exposure on the developing brain and consequent impairment, alternative explanations, including shared vulnerability factors that account for both adolescent cannabis use and negative psychosocial outcomes, have been proposed. Unfortunately, the number of causally informative studies considering adolescent cannabis and long-term psychosocial outcomes in adulthood is critically lacking, meaning that the potential mechanisms underlying these associations remain to be explicated. The few existing causally informative studies do suggest that adolescent cannabis use may be causally associated with poorer school performance, lower educational attainment, lower occupational prestige, and lower income in adulthood, even accounting for other shared vulnerability factors.

FUTURE DIRECTIONS

An extensive body of literature documenting research conducted over the past several decades establishes associations between adolescent cannabis use and impairment in important psychosocial domains in both adolescence and adulthood. We must now turn our attention to the mechanisms underlying these associations. Although it is not ethical to randomly assign adolescents to cannabis exposure, as in an experiment, the existing causally informative studies have provided important initial insights into potentially causal effects of cannabis exposure on psychosocial functioning. Additional causally informative research using epidemiologic samples and quasi-experimental designs are critical to move the field forward. One exciting future direction lies with the Adolescent Brain Cognitive Development (ABCD) study,[56] a multisite investigation of more than 11,000 children first assessed at age 9 or 10 years, who will be followed up every 6 months for 10 years, through adolescence, and holds considerable promise for mapping adolescent cannabis use and the developing addiction cycle. Critically, the ABCD study also includes more than 800 twin pairs, which, particularly in the context of its prospective, longitudinal study design, increases causal inference considerably.[57] Of note, although adolescence and the transition into emerging adulthood is an optimal time for investigations of cannabis initiation and use and misuse, there is also great potential value in even earlier investigations, such as the recently launched Healthy Brain and Child Development (HBCD) study,[58] as the risk processes that lead some adolescents to initiate cannabis use earlier or misuse cannabis were in place years earlier, indexed by familial and contextual adversities and early-evident individual differences in behavioral disinhibition. Considered together, existing research suggests delineating the developmental origins of cannabis use to identify the earliest causal risk factors and maximize early prevention efforts will promote adaptive psychosocial functioning in adolescence and adulthood.

CLINICS CARE POINTS

- Adolescent cannabis use is associated with psychosocial impairment in a range of important domains of functioning, including interpersonal relationships, socioeconomic status, and legal domains

- To date, very few causally informative studies have been conducted, meaning mechanistic links between adolescent cannabis use and long-term psychosocial functioning in adulthood remain unclear

- Causally informative studies suggest a potential causal effect of cannabis exposure on adult socioeconomic outcomes

- Clinicians working with adolescents using cannabis should be aware of individual and contextual vulnerability factors that might lead to negative psychosocial functioning outcomes, even with the successful cessation of cannabis use

ACKNOWLEDGMENTS

Research reported in this article was supported by the National Institute on Drug Abuse and the National Institute of Mental Health of the National Institutes of Health-under award numbers U01DA041120 (S. Wilson) and T32MH015755 (J.D. Schaefer).

DISCLOSURE

The authors have nothing to disclose.

REFERENCES

1. Gómez-López M, Viejo C, Ortega-Ruiz R. Well-being and romantic relationships: a systematic review in adolescence and emerging adulthood. Int J Environ Res Public Health 2019;16(13):2415.
2. Mitic M, Woodcock K, Amering M, et al. Toward an integrated model of supportive peer relationships in early adolescence: a systematic review and exploratory meta-analysis. Front Psychol 2020;12:589403.
3. Gliksberg O, Livne O, Lev-Ran S, et al. The association between cannabis use and perceived social support: the mediating role of decreased social network. Int J Ment Health Addict 2021. https://doi.org/10.1007/s11469-021-00549-4.
4. Li Y, Guo G. Heterogeneous peer effects on marijuana use: evidence from a natural experiment. Soc Sci Med 2020;252:112907.
5. Moriarty J, McVicar D, Higgins K. Cross-section and panel estimates of peer effects in early adolescent cannabis use: with a little help from my 'friends once removed. Soc Sci Med 2016;163:37–44.
6. Pérez A, Ariza C, Sánchez-Martínez F, et al. Cannabis consumption initiation among adolescents: a longitudinal study. Addict Behav 2010;35(2):129–34.
7. Brook JS, Balka EB, Whiteman M. The risks for late adolescence of early adolescent marijuana use. Am J Public Health 1999;89(10):1549–54.
8. Fergusson DM, Horwood LJ. Early onset cannabis use and psychosocial adjustment in young adults. Addiction 1997;92(3):279–96.
9. Chan GCK, Becker D, Butterworth P, et al. Young-adult compared to adolescent onset of regular cannabis use: a 20-year prospective cohort study of later consequences. Drug Alcohol Rev 2021;40(4):627–36.
10. Fergusson DM, Boden JM. Cannabis use and later life outcomes. Addiction 2008; 103(6):969–76.
11. Agrawal A, Few L, Nelson EC, et al. Adolescent cannabis use and repeated voluntary unprotected sex in women: cannabis and risky sex in women. Addiction 2016;111(11):2012–20.
12. Longmore, M. A., Manning, W. D., & Giordano, P. C. (2013). Parent-child relationships in adolescence.
13. Branstetter SA, Furman W. Buffering effect of parental monitoring knowledge and parent-adolescent relationships on consequences of adolescent substance use. J Child Fam Stud 2013;22(2):192–8.
14. Vermeulen-Smit E, Verdurmen JEE, Engels R, et al. The role of general parenting and cannabis-specific parenting practices in adolescent cannabis and other illicit drug use. Drug Alcohol Depend 2015;147:222–8.
15. Chan GC, Kelly AB, Carroll A, et al. Peer drug use and adolescent polysubstance use: do parenting and school factors moderate this association? Addict Behav 2017;64:78–81.

16. Jackson D, Mannix J. Then suddenly he went right off the rails: mothers' stories of adolescent cannabis use. Contemp Nurse 2003;14(2):169–79.

17. Usher K, Jackson D, O'Brien L. Shattered dreams: parental experiences of adolescent substance abuse. Int J Ment Health Nurs 2007;16(6):422–30.

18. Brook JS, Lee JY, Finch SJ, et al. The association of externalizing behavior and parent–child relationships: an intergenerational study. J Child Fam Stud 2012; 21(3):418–27.

19. Fairbairn CE, Briley DA, Kang D, et al. A meta-analysis of longitudinal associations between substance use and interpersonal attachment security. Psychol Bull 2018;144(5):532–55.

20. Lorenzetti V, Hoch E, Hall W. Adolescent cannabis use, cognition, brain health and educational outcomes: a review of the evidence. Eur Neuropsychopharmacol 2020;36:169–80.

21. Macleod J, Oakes R, Copello A, et al. Psychological and social sequelae of cannabis and other illicit drug use by young people: a systematic review of longitudinal, general population studies. Lancet 2004;363(9421):1579–88.

22. Townsend L, Flisher AJ, King G. A systematic review of the relationship between high school dropout and substance use. Clin Child Fam Psychol Rev 2007;10(4): 295–317.

23. Horwood LJ, Fergusson DM, Hayatbakhsh MR, et al. Cannabis use and educational achievement: findings from three Australasian cohort studies. Drug Alcohol Depend 2010;110(3):247–53.

24. Lee JY, Brook JS, Finch SJ, et al. Trajectories of marijuana use from adolescence to adulthood predicting unemployment in the mid 30s. Am J Addict 2015;24(5): 452–9.

25. Thompson K, Leadbeater B, Ames M, et al. Associations between marijuana use trajectories and educational and occupational success in young adulthood. Prev Sci 2019;20(2):257–69.

26. Zhang C, Brook JS, Leukefeld CG, et al. Trajectories of marijuana use from adolescence to adulthood as predictors of unemployment status in the early forties. Am J Addict 2016;25(3):203–9.

27. Airagnes G, Lemogne C, Meneton P, et al. Alcohol, tobacco and cannabis use are associated with job loss at follow-up: findings from the CONSTANCES cohort. PLoS One 2019;14(9):e0222361.

28. Boden JM, Lee JO, Horwood LJ, et al. Modelling possible causality in the associations between unemployment, cannabis use, and alcohol misuse. Soc Sci Med 2017;175:127–34.

29. Okechukwu CA, Molino J, Soh Y. Associations between marijuana use and involuntary job loss in the United States: representative longitudinal and cross-sectional samples. J Occup Environ Med 2019;61(1):21–8.

30. Popovici I, French MT. Cannabis use, employment, and income: fixed-effects analysis of panel data. J Behav Health Serv Res 2014;41(2):185–202.

31. Braun BL, Hannan P, Wolfson M, et al. Occupational attainment, smoking, alcohol intake, and marijuana use: ethnic-gender differences in the CARDIA study. Addict Behav 2000;25(3):399–414.

32. Schuster C, O'Malley PM, Bachman JG, et al. Adolescent marijuana use and adult occupational attainment: a longitudinal study from age 18 to 28. Subst Use Misuse 2001;36(8):997–1014.

33. Beverly HK, Castro Y, Opara I. Age of first marijuana use and its impact on education attainment and employment status. J Drug Issues 2019;49(2):228–37.

34. Fergusson DM, Lynskey MT, Horwood LJ. Factors associated with continuity and changes in disruptive behavior patterns between childhood and adolescence. J Abnormal Child Psychol 1996;24(5):533–53.

35. Newcomb MD, Bentler PM. Impact of adolescent drug use and social support on problems of young adults: a longitudinal study. J Abnormal Psychol 1988; 97(1):64.

36. Hall W, Leung J, Lynskey M. The effects of cannabis use on the development of adolescents and young adults. Annu Rev Dev Psychol 2020;2:461–83.

37. Iacono WG, Malone SM, McGue M. Behavioral disinhibition and the development of early-onset addiction: common and specific influences. Annu Rev Clin Psychol 2008;4:325–48.

38. Adinoff B, Reiman A. Implementing social justice in the transition from illicit to legal cannabis. Am J Drug Alcohol Abuse 2019;45(6):673–88.

39. Van den Bergh O, Walentynowicz M. Accuracy and bias in retrospective symptom reporting. Curr Opin Psychiatry 2016;29(5):302–8.

40. Chye Y, Christensen E, Yücel M. Cannabis use in adolescence: a review of neuroimaging findings. J Dual Diagn 2020;16(1):83–105.

41. Nader DA, Sanchez ZM. Effects of regular cannabis use on neurocognition, brain structure, and function: a systematic review of findings in adults. Am J Drug Alcohol Abuse 2018;44(1):4–18.

42. Gobbi G, Atkin T, Zytynski T, et al. Association of cannabis use in adolescence and risk of depression, anxiety, and suicidality in young adulthood: a systematic review and meta-analysis. JAMA Psychiatry 2019;76(4):426–34.

43. Lac A, Luk JW. Testing the amotivational syndrome: marijuana use longitudinally predicts lower self-efficacy even after controlling for demographics, personality, and alcohol and cigarette use. Prev Sci 2018;19(2):117–26.

44. Levine A, Clemenza K, Rynn M, et al. Evidence for the risks and consequences of adolescent cannabis exposure. J Am Acad Child Adolesc Psychiatry 2017;56(3): 214–25.

45. Mills R, Kisely S, Alati R, et al. Child maltreatment and cannabis use in young adulthood: a birth cohort study. Addiction 2017;112(3):494–501.

46. Peters EN, Bae D, Barrington-Trimis JL, et al. Prevalence and sociodemographic correlates of adolescent use and polyuse of combustible, vaporized, and edible cannabis products. JAMA Netw Open 2018;1(5). https://doi.org/10.1001/jamanetworkopen.2018.2765.

47. McGue M, Osler M, Christensen K. Causal inference and observational research: the utility of twins. Perspect Psychol Sci 2010;5:546–56.

48. Rutter M. Proceeding from observed correlation to causal inference: the use of natural experiments. Perspect Psychol Sci 2007;2(4):377–95.

49. Leonard KE, Eiden RD. Marital and family processes in the context of alcohol use and alcohol disorders. Annu Rev Clin Psychol 2007;3:285–310.

50. Marshal MP. For better or for worse? The effects of alcohol use on marital functioning. Clin Psychol Rev 2003;23(7):959–97.

51. Gillespie NA, Zhu G, Neale MC, et al. Direction of causation modeling between cross-sectional measures of parenting and psychological distress in female twins. Behav Genet 2003;33(4):383–96.

52. Grant JD, Lynskey MT, Scherrer JF, et al. A cotwin-control analysis of drug use and abuse/dependence risk associated with early-onset cannabis use. Addict Behav 2010;35(1):35–41.

53. Verweij KJH, Huizink AC, Agrawal A, et al. Is the relationship between early-onset cannabis use and educational attainment causal or due to common liability? Drug Alcohol Depend 2013;133(2). https://doi.org/10.1016/j.drugalcdep.2013.07.034.
54. Schaefer JD, Hamdi NR, Malone SM, et al. Associations between adolescent cannabis use and young-adult functioning in three longitudinal twin studies. Proc Natl Acad Sci U S A 2021;118(14). e2013180118.
55. Marie O, Zölitz U. High" achievers? Cannabis access and academic performance. Rev Econ Stud 2017;84(3):1210–37.
56. Jernigan TL, Brown SA. Introduction. Dev Cogn Neurosci 2018;32:1–3.
57. Iacono WG, Heath AC, Hewitt JK, et al. The utility of twins in developmental cognitive neuroscience research: how twins strengthen the ABCD research design. Dev Cogn Neurosci 2017;32:30–42.
58. Volkow ND, Gordon JA, Freund MP. The Healthy brain and child development study—shedding light on opioid exposure, COVID-19, and health disparities. JAMA Psychiatry 2021;78(5):471–2.

Adolescent Cannabis Use, Comorbid Attention-Deficit/ Hyperactivity Disorder, and Other Internalizing and Externalizing Disorders

Karla Molinero, MD[a], Jesse D. Hinckley, MD, PhD[b],*

KEYWORDS

- Adolescence • Anxiety • Attention-deficit/hyperactivity disorder (ADHD) • Cannabis
- Conduct disorder • Depression • Externalizing symptoms

KEY POINTS

- There are multiple potential negative consequences of cannabis use during adolescence including cognitive impairments in IQ, working memory, inhibition, and reasoning despite the increasing social acceptance of its use.
- Internalizing symptoms and disorders including depression and anxiety are highly comorbid with cannabis use and cannabis use disorder while attention-deficit/hyperactivity disorder (ADHD) and other externalizing symptoms and behaviors may be risk factors for them.
- The overlap of symptoms observed in chronic cannabis use and ADHD poses significant diagnostic challenges and may interfere with pharmacologic management of ADHD.
- Psychosocial interventions for ADHD including behavioral management and training interventions have the potential to be adapted for the management of comorbid substance use, internalizing, and other externalizing disorders.
- Understanding longitudinally the differences between internalizing and externalizing symptoms/disorders and the correlation with subsequent substance use can be used to direct preventative interventions to higher risk individuals.

This article originally appeared in *Child and Adolescent Psychiatric Clinics*, Volume 32 Issue 1, January 2023.
[a] Department of Psychiatry, University of Colorado School of Medicine, 1890 N Revere Court, MS-F570, Aurora, CO 80045, USA; [b] Division of Addiction Science, Treatment, and Prevention, Department of Psychiatry, University of Colorado School of Medicine, 1890 North Revere Court, MS-F570, Aurora, CO 80045, USA
* Corresponding author.
E-mail address: jesse.hinckley@cuanschutz.edu

Psychiatr Clin N Am 46 (2023) 691–702
https://doi.org/10.1016/j.psc.2023.03.007   **psych.theclinics.com**

INTRODUCTION

Cannabis use is a growing area of concern for pediatric mental health given the ongoing neurodevelopment throughout children and adolescents. Negative consequences of cannabis use during this vulnerable period include cognitive impairments in IQ, working memory, inhibition, and reasoning.[1] Despite the adverse effects and long-term outcomes from cannabis use, individuals continue to seek its primary intoxicating or euphoric effects of feeling "high." Adolescents have reported reasons for ongoing use to include euphoric effects, means of coping, and social cohesion.[2] Additionally, some individuals who use cannabis cite temporary relief from symptoms of anxiety, depression, and pain as a motivation for continued use.[3]

Adolescents aged 12 to 18 years who use cannabis at least twice a month for 6 months or longer are also at increased risk for poor academic performance, delinquent behavior, psychiatric problems, and arrests.[4] Further, cannabis use is associated with poorer mental health outcomes, and comorbid mental health disorders are associated with problematic cannabis use.[2,5] Individuals who use cannabis may experience more severe and persistent depression and anxiety, as well as worse cannabis withdrawal and cravings.[5] Among individuals with major depressive disorder (MDD), cannabis use has been associated with decreased quality of life, reduced efficacy of pharmacologic treatments, and poorer daily functioning.[6] Although the biologic cause and directionality of comorbid disorders remains unclear, it is vital to accurately diagnose and manage these co-occurring disorders.[7]

One notable clinical challenge is the diagnosis and management of comorbid attention-deficit/hyperactivity disorder (ADHD) and cannabis use disorder (CUD). Soler Artigas and colleagues reviewed summary statistics in meta-analyses studying the relationship between ADHD and substance use and found cannabis was the most used among these youth.[8] Problematic cannabis use and ADHD exhibit overlapping signs and symptoms and may result in similar academic and behavioral challenges.[9] Other mental health disorders are often present in adolescents with problematic cannabis use and ADHD. Further, adolescents commonly endorsed 2 or more psychiatric syndromes when entering treatment of cannabis use. The most common internalizing disorders are depression and anxiety, with conduct disorder (CD) and oppositional defiant disorder being the most common externalizing disorders.[10]

Due to the interconnectedness of these various disorders, a well-developed breadth of clinical interventions including both pharmacologic and psychosocial becomes essential. Although the cause of comorbid disorders, including ADHD and CUD, is not well understood, clinicians face the challenge of diagnosing and managing these co-occurring disorders. The purpose of this article is to provide a greater understanding of the insights into the complex nature of cannabis use, ADHD, and comorbid internalizing and externalizing disorders to serve as guidance for the management of an often undertreated population.

ATTENTION-DEFICIT/HYPERACTIVITY DISORDER

ADHD is common, with a prevalence of approximately 4 million among school-aged youth in the United States.[8] Youth meeting criteria for ADHD demonstrate behavioral deficits in attention, self-regulation, and social competence and higher rates of executive functioning deficits including processing speed and working memory. ADHD is classified as a neurodevelopmental disorder, with symptoms typically present in early childhood. However, for numerous reasons (eg, access to care, adaptive functioning), many children go undiagnosed until adolescence. Further, CUD is common among youth with ADHD, with an estimated prevalence of 33% to 38%.[11] Research has suggested that individuals with ADHD are 7.9 times more likely to use cannabis than non-ADHD peers.[8] Both CUD and ADHD are independently associated with academic challenges, including disruptive classroom behavior, learning, and time management difficulties, often resulting in poor grades.[9] These overlapping cognitive deficits and social-behavioral challenges highlight the clinical importance of better understanding the intersectionality of these 2 populations to inform treatment planning and interventions. Early diagnosis of ADHD before the initiation of cannabis use may also reduce potential long-term problems associated with these co-occurring disorders.

The significant symptom overlap of chronic cannabis use and ADHD poses significant diagnostic challenges. Initiation of cannabis use before the diagnosis of ADHD may result in more pronounced maladaptive effects of cannabis than non-ADHD peers.[11] There is also interest in understanding the shared biology of ADHD and problematic cannabis use. The individual heritability factors of ADHD and cannabis use initiation have been observed to be between 70% and 80% and 40% and 48%, respectively.[8] There are also significant overlapping features of the neurocircuitry implicated in both problematic cannabis use and ADHD, including dysfunction in frontal cortical regions responsible for executive functioning and response inhibition, and the dopaminergic reward systems.[8,12] Chronic cannabis use is associated with hyperactivation of frontal cortical regions, which impairs working memory and contributes to deficits in executive functioning similar to those found in ADHD.[13] Thus, differentiating the neurocognitive deficits of problematic cannabis use and ADHD may not be feasible or practical.

In addition, societal perception of cannabis use and its harmful effects have evolved during the past few decades.[14] There is growing perceptions of its therapeutic use and decreased perceived harm or deviance. These changes in perception become increasingly important among youth with ADHD, who have an earlier age of onset of substance use and increased likelihood for developing a substance use disorder (SUD).[15] Many adolescents think that cannabis improves their ADHD symptoms or remedies side effects from stimulant medications, whereas the potential risks and interactions from combining cannabis and stimulants are often not considered.[16] Yet, those individuals with hyperactive/impulsive symptoms may be at a higher risk for cannabis misuse or dependence given a self-medication function while those with inattentive subtype of ADHD may actually experience worsening symptoms.[16] Further, ADHD symptoms are correlated with greater severity of cannabis cravings and associated with greater risk of relapse.[11] For clinicians, it becomes even more challenging to circumvent the societal normalization of cannabis despite a growing literature of associated poor health outcomes.

INTERNALIZING SYMPTOMS AND DISORDERS

Youth with ADHD experience increased social and emotional deficits,[17] which limits availability of coping resources and increases the risk of experiencing anxiety and depression (**Box 1**). Family history of depression and anxiety is further associated with increased risk of internalizing symptoms and disorders. Approximately 13% to 51% of youth with ADHD have comorbid internalizing disorders and 25% of youth with ADHD exhibit an anxiety disorder.[18] Longitudinal studies estimate up to 50% of individuals with predominantly ADHD inattentive type have an anxiety disorder, which often goes undiagnosed.[18] Given the high prevalence of comorbidity, understanding the developmental pathway of ADHD and anxiety is important. Overlapping symptoms in ADHD and anxiety disorders include restlessness, irritability, difficulty concentrating, and sleep disturbance. The term "anxiety" relates to worry, separation fears,

---

Box 1
Attention-deficit/hyperactivity disorder and comorbid internalizing/externalizing disorders

- Symptoms of cannabis withdrawal can resemble internalizing symptoms for up to 2 weeks following cessation and should be considered before diagnosis of a mood or anxiety disorder.
- Social and emotional deficits of ADHD increase risk for comorbid internalizing symptoms and disorders.
- Thorough evaluation for anxiety disorders should be completed in an adolescent presenting with a concern for ADHD to avoid possible misdiagnosis.
- Externalizing disorders and early onset of symptoms in childhood are associated with increased risk of substance use.
- Greater severity of ADHD symptoms is associated with increased delinquent behaviors.

---

and obsessive thoughts, which are not core features of ADHD. In youth with ADHD, subsequent anxiety disorders may also arise from a collection of failure experiences related to ADHD deficits that contribute to chronic fear and worry.[18] Further, "anxious impulsivity" may present as restless behavior that is misinterpreted as hyperactivity.[18] Considering the interrelatedness of symptomatology and high rates of comorbidity, it becomes important to screen for anxiety disorders and develop a thorough timeline of symptoms to inform treatment planning and monitor clinical progression.

Adolescents and young adults with ADHD also frequently report significant sleep disturbances, which are not well understood. Individuals with ADHD are 3 times more likely to have circadian rhythm sleep disturbances as well as longer sleep-onset latencies.[19–24] This typically manifests in a variety of ways, including shifts in sleep patterns with inability to fall asleep and difficulty staying asleep or waking up early.[20–22] Poor sleep can then yield increased mood and cognitive problems, as well as fatigue and exhaustion, which may exacerbate symptoms of depression, anxiety, and ADHD.[19,21,22]

The relationship between cannabis use and internalizing symptoms and disorders has also been a focus of research and clinical interest (see **Box 1**). The symptomatology of these disorders includes depression, anxiety, somatic features, traumatic distress, and suicide.[10] Although problematic cannabis use is often associated with worsening symptoms of internalizing disorders, direction of the relationship or causality is unknown.[25] Further, studies have shown internalizing symptoms associated with ADHD are also risk factors for problematic substance use.[23,24] Internalizing disorders may also be a moderator of ADHD-related risk for developing problematic substance use and subsequent SUD and are associated with prolonged course of illness.[10] However, the effect of internalizing symptoms on an individual's well-being tends to be the primary reason treatment is sought among those with problematic cannabis use, rather than the substance use itself.[10]

The directionality of relationships between cannabis use with mood disorders and anxiety disorders continues to be obscure. Studies have found rates of comorbid MDD and generalized anxiety disorder to be 3 times higher among those with CUD.[13,26] Cannabis use is also associated with higher rates of lifetime MDD and suicide attempt.[23] It is valuable to understand the discontinuation or sudden reduction of cannabis use can lead to withdrawal that may mimic internalizing symptoms and occur one to 2 days after the last use and can last up to 2 weeks if heavy use. It is not uncommon for youth to have limited resources to maintain a constant supply of cannabis and may have recurrent periods of withdrawal that can present with anxiety or nervousness, restlessness, irritability, anger, fatigue, dysphoria, depressed mood, decreased appetite, amotivation, and sleep difficulty. In fewer cases, suicidal ideation, nightmares, and strange dreams may also occur.[27] If there are comorbid anxiety and depressive disorders, withdrawal periods may exacerbate those symptoms and complicate the diagnostic assessment.

EXTERNALIZING SYMPTOMS AND DISORDERS

There is a rather complex relationship between ADHD, CD, and SUD risk. Both ADHD and CD are independent risk factors for the development of an SUD.[28,29] A common predisposing factor may be the general disinhibitory behavioral processes (ie, hyperactivity/impulsivity), which are features of both ADHD and CD.[28] One study found youth with ADHD were also 4 to 5 times more likely to progress to heavy cigarette and cannabis use compared with youth without ADHD.[30] Further, children with persistent and worsening delinquent behaviors were shown to be at higher risk for problematic substance use.[31] When disruptive behaviors and high conflict occur primarily within the family or with parents, these youth were more likely to engage in heavier substance use in late adolescence when compared with youth without high levels of conflict.[30] Understanding patterns of symptom progression and quality of parent–child relationships may provide insight into the likelihood of an SUD developing and play a direct role on the escalation of overall risk behavior.

Externalizing disorders, particularly CD and related behaviors, in individuals with ADHD have also been investigated as risk factors for substance use. A recent meta-analysis found the odds of perpetrating violence was 2.01 to 2.62 times higher among adolescents who use cannabis compared with adolescents who do not, with the highest odds among persistent heavy users (OR = 2.81, 95% CI 1.26–3.23).[32] The cognitive effects of cannabis that may contribute to the risk of behavioral dysregulation include impaired ability to reduce aggressive impulses, anxiety or panic, feelings of paranoia, and increased arousal.[32] Symptoms related to disruptive disorders of childhood, personality traits related to behavioral disinhibition, and traits of CD were also negatively correlated with constraint adherence and traditional moral values while positively correlated to impulsive thrill-seeking behaviors.[28,33] A history of abuse and maltreatment, poor parental monitoring/involvement, affiliation with deviant peers, and weak attachment to their schools have also been associated with disruptive behaviors.[28] Cumulative exposure to multiple risks is hypothesized to contribute to externalizing disorders in youth and subsequent problematic substance use.[28]

TREATMENT
Pharmacologic Management

Pharmacologic management of ADHD includes stimulant and nonstimulant medications, with stimulant medications typically considered first line.[34–36] A recent meta-analysis establishing evidence to support the use of extended-release methylphenidate and amphetamine formulations, atomoxetine, and extended-release guanfacine for the treatment of noncomorbid ADHD in adolescents.[35] Although treatment of ADHD improves academic, economic, and social outcomes, less is known about the efficacy of pharmacologic management of ADHD among youth with comorbid CUD.[37,38] Treatment providers might insist the youth be abstinent before treating comorbid mental health conditions. They may also be hesitant to use particularly psychostimulant medications in these youth. Because cannabis is also associated with executive dysfunction, including impairments of attention and working memory, it is unclear if ADHD medications will be effective if the youth is still using cannabis. There may also be concerns about misuse and diversion of psychostimulants by adolescents with CUD, although few studies may begin to address these clinical concerns.

Stimulant medications

To date, 2 randomized controlled trials (RCTs) have investigated long-acting formulations of methylphenidate (MPH-SODAS and OROS-MPH) in adolescents with ADHD and SUDs. In a randomized, placebo-controlled crossover study design, Szobot and colleagues evaluated MPH-SODAS in adolescents with ADHD and comorbid cannabis use (N = 16, 100% male), 43.8% of whom also used cocaine.[39] Participants had greater reductions in ADHD symptoms when taking MPH compared with placebo, although there was no significant change in substance use. Riggs and colleagues subsequently completed a multisite RCT of osmotic-release methylphenidate (OROS-MPH) combined with cognitive behavioral therapy (CBT) in adolescents with ADHD and comorbid SUD (N = 303, 79% male, 66.7% cannabis dependence, and 29.7% alcohol dependence).[40] Adolescents in both the OROS-MPH and placebo groups showed clinically significant improvements in ADHD and substance use, although no significant between-group differences were found. Although the effectiveness of OROS-MPH versus placebo was unclear, parents reported significantly lower ADHD symptoms in adolescents in the OROS-MPH group, and these adolescents showed significant improvements in problem-solving ability and acquisition of focused coping skills compared with the placebo group. Overall, OROS-MPH was relatively well tolerated. Adolescents who use cannabis more frequently (>40% of days) were more likely to report side effects from OROS-MPH, although no specific side effect and no serious adverse drug events were associated with cannabis use.[41] Of note, a recent study by Skoglund and colleagues found individuals with ADHD and comorbid SUD typically require higher doses of methylphenidate compared with individuals without SUD and postulated that lack of efficacy may be due to inadequate dosing.[42]

To investigate the risk of misuse and diversion of OROS-MPH among adolescents with ADHD and comorbid SUD, Winhusen and colleagues analyzed these outcomes by baseline substance use severity.[41] Cannabis and tobacco were the most frequently used substances (11/28 days and 24/28 days, respectively). There were higher subjective ratings of effectiveness of the medication (P<.001) and feeling high (P<.01) but not in craving the medication (P = .18) or craving substances (P = .06) among youth who received OROS-MPH. However, neither cannabis use nor substance use severity was significantly associated with misuse or diversion. Further, studies have shown that pharmacologic treatment of ADHD does not seem to increase the risk for developing a SUD.[43] Treatment of ADHD and comorbid substance use may also reduce the risk of alcohol and substance use ADHD[44] and may prevent the development or progression of SUD in adolescence and young adulthood.[45] In adults with ADHD, an RCT of extended-release mixed amphetamine salts found a significant decrease in the proportion of participants using cannabis over time, compared with placebo.[12] Thus, research suggests that treatment with a stimulant medication serves as a protective factor for substance use. Nonetheless, stimulant medications do have potential to be misused or abused, with a risk of diversion, particularly in unstructured or unsupervised settings,[46] which may be mitigated with parental involvement and close clinical follow-up.

Nonstimulant medications

Three nonstimulant medications have been investigated in small studies of adolescents with ADHD and comorbid substance use: atomoxetine, bupropion, and guanfacine.[37] Thurstone and colleagues completed a single-site RCT of atomoxetine versus placebo, combined with motivational interviewing and CBT in both groups for adolescents with ADHD and comorbid SUD.[47] Both treatment groups demonstrated improvements in ADHD scores and the number of days nonnicotine substances were used, with no significant between-group differences.

In 2 small studies of bupropion, Riggs and colleagues (N = 13, 100% male) and Solhkhah and colleagues (N = 14, 64% male) found adolescents with comorbid substance use tolerated bupropion well, with high medication compliance (85% and 90%, respectively).[48,49] In both studies, there was significant reduction in clinician-rated ADHD symptoms from baseline. The study by Riggs and colleagues was conducted in a residential substance use program, where all adolescents received substance use programming; no substance use outcomes were reported. In the study by Solhkhah and colleagues, 57% of participants received some form of counseling or psychotherapy, with significant reductions in substance abuse at the 6-month endpoint compared with baseline.

Although guanfacine has shown promising results in a 6-day preclinical trial,[50] its efficacy as a treatment option for adolescents with ADHD and comorbid cannabis use remains unknown.

Psychosocial Interventions

To date, no psychosocial interventions have been studied specifically for adolescents with ADHD and comorbid CUD. However, several psychosocial interventions for ADHD show potential to be adapted for the management of comorbid SUD, including CUD.[9,45] Psychosocial interventions for ADHD are broadly categorized as behavioral management or training interventions.[9,35] Behavioral management often uses selective reinforcement to enhance desired behaviors and selective ignoring to decrease problematic behaviors.[35] Conversely, training interventions are skills-based programs that can be implemented in a variety of settings, including clinic and school. Training interventions may also incorporate family components to optimize the home environment and provide behavioral management.

Box 2
Best practices for attention-deficit/hyperactivity disorder and comorbid cannabis use

- Conduct a thorough diagnostic assessment, including comorbid mental health and substance use disorders, academic functioning and learning, and family functioning.

- Build a strong treatment alliance through acknowledging the youth's goals, values, and role in shared decision-making.

- Engage adolescents in motivational interviewing and provide brief intervention as indicated in response to comorbid substance use.

- Integrate management of ADHD and comorbid substance use using therapeutic approaches and medications as indicated.

- When determining whether to prescribe a medication, consider degree of impairment caused by ADHD.

- When prescribing psychostimulants, use long-acting forms on a scheduled dosing regimen (avoid "as needed" dosing) and monitor compliance and diversion.

- For individuals assessed to be at high-risk of diversion or misuse, consider nonstimulant medications and therapy options as first-line.

- For adolescents with severe substance use disorders, consider referral to substance-specific treatment programs.

Family-focused psychoeducation models have been proven to be helpful for youths with ADHD by increasing medication and behavioral treatment effects and adherence.[9] Peer programs further provide an opportunity for youth with ADHD to improve social skills, promote social competence, and reduce the risk of peer rejection.[24] These models have shown a direct positive effect on ADHD symptoms and overall prosocial functioning.[9]

Considering the clinical trials by Riggs and colleagues and Thurstone and colleagues, integration of therapy targeting substance use may also be effective for the management of substance use and comorbid mental health disorders, including ADHD.[40,47] In these studies, the authors postulated the lack of between-group differences between atomoxetine or OROS-MPH and placebo may be due to the impact of the background CBT treatment received by both groups. Although not specific to ADHD, such therapeutic interventions, including motivational enhancement therapy (MET) combined with CBT (MET/CBT) and the Adolescent-Community Reinforcement Approach, may be more broadly applicable in adolescent mental health treatment programs.[51,52]

SUMMARY

Concern about cannabis use among youth has become more prevalent during the past decades as access and social acceptance of it have increased. Problematic substance use rarely presents on its own in adolescence and frequently co-occurs with ADHD, as well as other internalizing and externalizing disorders. Individually these disorders can be challenging to treat, and comorbid ADHD and CUD are associated with a greater symptom burden and treatment complexity. Approaching treatment planning with a biopsychosocial perspective can allow for a better understanding of the interconnectedness of these disorders. Although limited, evidence to date posits the standard of care should be comanagement of these disorders to improve outcomes and maximize the likelihood of adequate management or remission of both disorders.[7,46] Consideration of studies of pharmacologic and psychosocial interventions in adolescents with ADHD and CUD support an integrated approach for managing these comorbid disorders (**Box 2**).

CLINICS CARE POINTS

- As with youth who do not have comorbid substance use, ADHD should be diagnosed clinically through client, parent/guardian, and teacher report. Standardized screening tools for ADHD may be utilized in youth with comorbid substance use disorders

- When establishing confidentiality expectations with the client and family, the clinician should encourage the youth to discuss substance use with parents/guardians and inform the client and family that any urgent safety concerns regarding substance use (drinking and driving, high-risk use of opioids, etc.) will be disclosed to parents/guardians

- All youth with ADHD should be screened for current substance use, followed by brief intervention and diagnostic assessment as indicated by screening results, as well as screening for other internalizing (depression, anxiety) and externalizing problems

- Assessment of cannabis-related problems in youth with ADHD should include social relationships, self-esteem, motivation and productivity, academics, physical health, memory impairment, and legal problems

- Engage the youth with motivational interviewing to incorporate the youth's goals and motives into treatment planning

- When prescribing psychostimulants in youth with problematic cannabis use or cannabis use disorder, utilize long-acting formulations, use only scheduled (daily) doses and avoid "as needed" dosing, engage parents to monitor compliance and diversion, and routinely monitor for clinical changes in ADHD and substance use
- If the youth exhibits externalizing disorders and delinquent behaviors, evaluate family functioning and consider a referral for family-based therapies that incorporate parent training/support and behavioral modification stratregies

DISCLOSURE

Dr K. Molinero and Dr J.D. Hinckley have no relevant disclosures or conflicts of interest.

This work was funded by the National Institute on Drug Abuse grant number K12DA000357.

REFERENCES

1. Morin JG, Afzali MH, Bourque J, et al. A population-based analysis of the relationship between substance use and adolescent cognitive development. Am J Psychiatry 2019;176(2):98–106.
2. Mooney LJ, Zhu Y, Yoo C, et al. Reduction in cannabis use and functional status in physical health, mental health, and cognition. J Neuroimmune Pharmacol 2018; 13(4):479–87.
3. Sideli L, Trotta G, Spinazzola E, et al. Adverse effects of heavy cannabis use: even plants can harm the brain. Pain 2021;162(Suppl 1):S97–104.
4. Stanger C, Ryan SR, Scherer EA, et al. Clinic- and home-based contingency management plus parent training for adolescent cannabis use disorders. J Am Acad Child Adolesc Psychiatry 2015;54(6):445–53.e2.
5. Blader JC, Pliszka SR, Jensen PS, et al. Stimulant-responsive and stimulant-refractory aggressive behavior among children with ADHD. Pediatrics 2010; 126(4):e796–806.
6. Urits I, Gress K, Charipova K, et al. Cannabis use and its association with psychological disorders. Psychopharmacol Bull 2020;50(2):56–67.
7. Hinckley JD, Riggs P. Integrated treatment of adolescents with Co-occurring depression and substance use disorder. Child Adolesc Psychiatr Clin N Am 2019;28(3):461–72.
8. Soler Artigas M, Sanchez-Mora C, Rovira P, et al. Attention-deficit/hyperactivity disorder and lifetime cannabis use: genetic overlap and causality. Mol Psychiatry 2020;25(10):2493–503.
9. Hogue A, Evans SW, Levin FR. A Clinician's Guide to Co-occurring ADHD among adolescent substance users: comorbidity, neurodevelopmental risk, and evidence-based treatment options. J Child Adolesc Subst Abuse 2017;26(4): 277–92.
10. Chan YF, Dennis ML, Funk RR. Prevalence and comorbidity of major internalizing and externalizing problems among adolescents and adults presenting to substance abuse treatment. J Subst Abuse Treat 2008;34(1):14–24.
11. Mitchell JT, Sweitzer MM, Tunno AM, et al. I use weed for My ADHD": a Qualitative analysis of Online Forum discussions on cannabis use and ADHD. PLoS One 2016;11(5):e0156614.

12. Notzon DP, Mariani JJ, Pavlicova M, et al. Mixed-amphetamine salts increase abstinence from marijuana in patients with co-occurring attention-deficit/hyperactivity disorder and cocaine dependence. Am J Addict 2016;25(8):666–72.

13. Ferland JN, Hurd YL. Deconstructing the neurobiology of cannabis use disorder. Nat Neurosci 2020;23(5):600–10.

14. Hinckley J, Bhatia D, Ellingson J, et al. The impact of recreational cannabis legalization on youth: the Colorado experience. Eur Child Adolesc Psychiatry 2022. https://doi.org/10.1007/s00787-022-01981-0.

15. Mannuzza S, Klein RG, Truong NL, et al. Age of methylphenidate treatment initiation in children with ADHD and later substance abuse: prospective follow-up into adulthood. Am J Psychiatry 2008;165(5):604–9.

16. Loflin M, Earleywine M, De Leo J, et al. Subtypes of attention deficit-hyperactivity disorder (ADHD) and cannabis use. Subst Use Misuse 2014;49(4):427–34.

17. Faraone SV, Rostain AL, Blader J, et al. Practitioner Review: emotional dysregulation in attention-deficit/hyperactivity disorder - implications for clinical recognition and intervention. J Child Psychol Psychiatry 2019;60(2):133–50.

18. Jarrett MA, Ollendick TH. A conceptual review of the comorbidity of attention-deficit/hyperactivity disorder and anxiety: implications for future research and practice. Clin Psychol Rev 2008;28(7):1266–80.

19. Cortese S, Brown TE, Corkum P, et al. Assessment and management of sleep problems in youths with attention-deficit/hyperactivity disorder. J Am Acad Child Adolesc Psychiatry 2013;52(8):784–96.

20. Becker SP, Kapadia DK, Fershtman CEM, et al. Evening circadian preference is associated with sleep problems and daytime sleepiness in adolescents with ADHD. J Sleep Res 2020;29(1):e12936.

21. Arns M, JJS Kooij, Coogan AN. Review: identification and management of circadian rhythm sleep disorders as a transdiagnostic feature in child and adolescent psychiatry. J Am Acad Child Adolesc Psychiatry 2021;60(9):1085–95.

22. Zeron-Rugerio MF, Carpio-Arias TV, Ferreira-Garcia E, et al. ADHD subtypes are associated differently with circadian rhythms of motor activity, sleep disturbances, and body mass index in children and adolescents: a case-control study. Eur Child Adolesc Psychiatry 2021;30(12):1917–27.

23. Gobbi G, Atkin T, Zytynski T, et al. Association of cannabis use in adolescence and risk of depression, anxiety, and suicidality in young adulthood: a systematic review and meta-analysis. JAMA psychiatry 2019;76(4):426–34.

24. Vitulano ML, Fite PJ, Hopko DR, et al. Evaluation of underlying mechanisms in the link between childhood ADHD symptoms and risk for early initiation of substance use. Psychol Addict Behav 2014;28(3):816–27.

25. Farmer RF, Seeley JR, Kosty DB, et al. Internalizing and externalizing psychopathology as predictors of cannabis use disorder onset during adolescence and early adulthood. Psychol Addict Behav 2015;29(3):541–51.

26. Onaemo VN, Fawehinmi TO, D'Arcy C. Comorbid cannabis use disorder with major depression and generalized anxiety disorder: a systematic review with meta-analysis of Nationally Representative Epidemiological surveys. J Affect Disord 2021;281:467–75.

27. Zehra A, Burns J, Liu CK, et al. Cannabis addiction and the brain: a review. Focus (Am Psychiatr Publ) 2019;17(2):169–82.

28. Iacono WG, Malone SM, McGue M. Behavioral disinhibition and the development of early-onset addiction: common and specific influences. Annu Rev Clin Psychol 2008;4:325–48.

29. Howard AL, Molina BS, Swanson JM, et al. Developmental progression to early adult binge drinking and marijuana use from worsening versus stable trajectories of adolescent attention deficit/hyperactivity disorder and delinquency. Addiction 2015;110(5):784-95.
30. Sibley MH, Pelham WE, Molina BSG, et al. The role of early childhood ADHD and subsequent CD in the initiation and escalation of adolescent cigarette, alcohol, and marijuana use. J Abnorm Psychol 2014;123(2):362-74.
31. Howard AL, Kennedy TM, Macdonald EP, et al. Depression and ADHD-related risk for substance use in adolescence and early adulthood: Concurrent and prospective associations in the MTA. J Abnorm Child Psychol 2019;47(12):1903-16.
32. Dellazizzo L, Potvin S, Dou BY, et al. Association between the use of cannabis and physical violence in youths: a meta-Analytical investigation. Am J Psychiatry 2020;177(7):619-26.
33. Pingault JB, Cote SM, Galera C, et al. Childhood trajectories of inattention, hyperactivity and oppositional behaviors and prediction of substance abuse/dependence: a 15-year longitudinal population-based study. Mol Psychiatry 2013; 18(7):806-12.
34. Pliszka S, Issues AWGoQ. Practice parameter for the assessment and treatment of children and adolescents with attention-deficit/hyperactivity disorder. J Am Acad Child Adolesc Psychiatry 2007;46(7):894-921.
35. Chan E, Fogler JM, Hammerness PG. Treatment of attention-deficit/hyperactivity disorder in adolescents: a systematic review. JAMA 2016;315(18):1997-2008.
36. Drechsler R, Brem S, Brandeis D, et al. ADHD: current Concepts and treatments in children and adolescents. Neuropediatrics 2020;51(5):315-35.
37. Zaso MJ, Park A, Antshel KM. Treatments for adolescents with comorbid ADHD and substance use disorder: a systematic review. J Atten Disord 2020;24(9): 1215-26.
38. Hinckley J, Hopfer C. Marijuana legalization in Colorado: Increasing potency, changing risk perceptions, and emerging public health concerns for youth. Adolescent Psychiatry 2021;11(2):95-116.
39. Szobot CM, Rohde LA, Katz B, et al. A randomized crossover clinical study showing that methylphenidate-SODAS improves attention-deficit/hyperactivity disorder symptoms in adolescents with substance use disorder. Braz J Med Biol Res 2008;41(3):250-7.
40. Riggs PD, Winhusen T, Davies RD, et al. Randomized controlled trial of osmotic-release methylphenidate with cognitive-behavioral therapy in adolescents with attention-deficit/hyperactivity disorder and substance use disorders. J Am Acad Child Adolesc Psychiatry 2011;50(9):903-14.
41. Winhusen TM, Lewis DF, Riggs PD, et al. Subjective effects, misuse, and adverse effects of osmotic-release methylphenidate treatment in adolescent substance abusers with attention-deficit/hyperactivity disorder. J Child Adolesc Psychopharmacol 2011;21(5):455-63.
42. Skoglund C, Brandt L, D'Onofrio B, et al. Methylphenidate doses in Attention Deficit/Hyperactivity Disorder and comorbid substance use disorders. Eur Neuropsychopharmacol 2017;27(11):1144-52.
43. Wilens TE, Upadhyaya HP. Impact of substance use disorder on ADHD and its treatment. J Clin Psychiatry 2007;68(8):e20.
44. Hammerness P, Petty C, Faraone SV, et al. Do stimulants reduce the risk for alcohol and substance use in youth with ADHD? A secondary analysis of a prospective, 24-month open-Label study of osmotic-release methylphenidate. J Atten Disord 2017;21(1):71-7.

45. Ozgen H, Spijkerman R, Noack M, et al. Treatment of adolescents with Concurrent substance use disorder and attention-deficit/hyperactivity disorder: a systematic review. J Clin Med 2021;10(17).

46. Mariani JJ, Levin FR. Treatment strategies for co-occurring ADHD and substance use disorders. Am J Addict 2007;16(Suppl 1):45–54 [quiz: 55–6].

47. Thurstone C, Riggs PD, Salomonsen-Sautel S, et al. Randomized, controlled trial of atomoxetine for attention-deficit/hyperactivity disorder in adolescents with substance use disorder. J Am Acad Child Adolesc Psychiatry 2010;49(6):573–82.

48. Riggs PD, Leon SL, Mikulich SK, et al. An open trial of bupropion for ADHD in adolescents with substance use disorders and conduct disorder. J Am Acad Child Adolesc Psychiatry 1998;37(12):1271–8.

49. Solhkhah R, Wilens TE, Daly J, et al. Bupropion SR for the treatment of substance-abusing outpatient adolescents with attention-deficit/hyperactivity disorder and mood disorders. J Child Adolesc Psychopharmacol 2005;15(5):777–86.

50. Mathai DS, Holst M, Rodgman C, et al. Guanfacine Attenuates adverse effects of Dronabinol (THC) on working memory in adolescent-onset heavy cannabis users: a pilot study. J Neuropsychiatry Clin Neurosci 2018;30(1):66–76.

51. Brewer S, Godley MD, Hulvershorn LA. Treating mental health and substance use disorders in adolescents: what is on the Menu? Curr Psychiatry Rep 2017;19(1):5.

52. Godley SH, Smith JE, Passetti LL, et al. The Adolescent Community Reinforcement Approach (A-CRA) as a model paradigm for the management of adolescents with substance use disorders and co-occurring psychiatric disorders. Subst Abus 2014;35(4):352–63.

Cannabis and Psychosis

Michelle L. West, PhD*, Shadi Sharif, BA

KEYWORDS

- Cannabis • Psychosis • Adolescent • Youth • Early psychosis • Early intervention
- Clinical high risk • First-episode psychosis

KEY POINTS

- Psychosis and cannabis use overlap in young people.
- Research and clinical practice support several clinical considerations for understanding overlapping psychosis and cannabis use.
- Some research has investigated neurobiology of overlapping psychosis and cannabis use, but there are many unanswered questions.
- Clinical practice supports multiple treatment considerations for co-occurring psychosis and cannabis use, but there is limited clinical trial research investigating treatments.

PSYCHOSIS BACKGROUND

Psychosis is a cluster of symptoms that involve difficulties knowing what is real and what is not real. As with any mental health experience, psychosis can be seen as a spectrum of experiences (from absent, to normative or mild, to clinically significant, to acute or severe). Psychosis spectrum experiences are heterogenous and complex, so understanding them optimally involves gathering a comprehensive history and timeline to build a conceptualization.

Psychosis symptoms are commonly divided into two clusters: positive symptoms and negative symptoms. Positive symptoms are additions to typical human experience, including delusions, hallucinations, and disorganized speech and behavior. Delusions involve thought content (what thoughts and beliefs you have), sometimes defined as usual beliefs that a person holds with certainty despite contrary evidence. Some common types of delusions include paranoid/persecutory delusions (eg, that an entity wants to harm you), grandiose delusions (eg, that you have special powers or abilities), and delusions of influence (eg, that others can influence or control you). Hallucinations are defined as perceptions that occur without an external stimulus

This article originally appeared in *Child and Adolescent Psychiatric Clinics*, Volume 32 Issue 1, January 2023.

Department of Psychiatry, University of Colorado School of Medicine, Anschutz Health Sciences Building, 1890 N Revere Court, Mailstop F443, Aurora, CO 80045, USA

* Corresponding author.

E-mail address: michelle.west@cuanschutz.edu

(eg, when a person hears, sees, feels, tastes, or smells something that is not there). Disorganized speech is when a person struggles to communicate their thoughts in a way that other people can understand (eg, jumping from topic to topic, connecting thoughts illogically). Similarly, disorganized behavior involves ways in which a person's behavior may not match their current situation and can be confusing or concerning to observers (eg, laughing at inappropriate times, poor self-care).

On the other hand, negative symptoms are reductions to the typical human experience, including reduced motivation (amotivation), reduced intensity of emotional experience (feeling no emotions), reduced expression of emotions (eg, constricted or flat affect), social withdrawal (reduced contact with people or participation in social interactions), and decline in role functioning. Negative symptoms make it difficult for a person to experience pleasure and feel drive to execute daily tasks. Although positive symptoms tend to be more commonly known and recognized, negative symptoms are commonly associated with poorer treatment response and functioning.[1]

Although commonly associated with schizophrenia diagnosis, psychosis is not specific to one diagnosis. Psychotic symptoms may be transdiagnostic, meaning that they may occur in multiple mental health and other medical diagnoses. Mental health diagnoses that can involve experience of psychosis include (but are not limited to) major depressive disorder with psychotic features, schizophrenia, borderline personality disorder, bipolar disorder with psychotic features, and cannabis-induced psychotic disorder. In addition, psychosis can be experienced without meeting criteria for a mental health diagnosis (eg, a person may experience hallucinations that do not cause them distress or impairment). Although commonly associated with mental illness, psychosis spectrum experiences (particularly subthreshold or milder experiences) are far more common than people think. For instance, many people have experienced mild hallucinations, including hearing someone call your name but realizing no one was there.

PSYCHOSIS IN ADOLESCENTS

Adolescents may experience psychosis spectrum symptoms in a variety of ways, and research has tended to categorize these experiences under a few different labels. A first, although rare, example of how psychosis may present in young people is child-onset schizophrenia, which means that a child meets criteria for schizophrenia before the age of 10 years. Child-onset schizophrenia is uncommon, representing only 0.1% to 1% of all cases of schizophrenia.[2] Because of its early and typically rapid onset, child-onset schizophrenia generally involves more severe symptomatology.[3]

There is increasing emphasis on understanding and intervening in the early stages of developing psychosis. Clinical high risk for psychosis (CHR-p) is a term capturing experiences that suggest risk for developing psychosis. This phase typically occurs at ages 12 to 30 years but can happen outside this range. The most commonly identified signs of risk are attenuated (subthreshold) positive symptoms.[4] Subthreshold positive symptoms mean that a person is still able to question their experiences (ie, "insight" is intact) and are typically more intermittent. Research suggests that about 15% to 30% of young people who meet CHR-p criteria progress to developing acute psychosis.[5] Although many people at CHR-p never develop a full psychotic disorder and symptoms may resolve with time, CHR-p may be a risk phase for multiple mental health diagnoses so can develop into nonpsychotic diagnosis.[6] First-episode psychosis (FEP) refers to experiencing acute psychosis, in which a person loses the ability to question psychotic symptoms (loss of "insight"), for a clinically significant time. FEP usually occurs in mid-teens and early 20s, with a tendency for earlier onset in men than women.[7] Research investigating mental health needs of youth who identify them-selves as nonbinary or transgender is limited,[8,9] and there are no known estimates of age of onset for these young people. See **Table 1** for brief FEP and CHR-p case examples.

Most CHR-p research on subthreshold positive symptoms is in help-seeking young people and families, suggesting that these experiences cause distress or concern. However, research in community samples suggests that "psychosis-like experiences" may be even more common in young people than commonly believed. For example, one community sample of teenagers (ages 13 to 17 years) endorsed self-reported psy-chosis-like experiences at rates ranging from 10.9% to 91.5%.[10] Although infrequent psychosis-like experiences were common, frequent experiences were uncommon, suggesting that these experiences may be more clinically significant if they are begin-ning to happen regularly.

PREVALENCE OF CANNABIS USE IN EARLY PSYCHOSIS

Substance use (ranging from rare use, to casual use, to misuse) is prevalent in early psychosis, both in clinical high risk (CHR-p) and in FEP. Rates of substance use may vary between 22% and 50% of the young people with FEP, with cannabis as the most prevalent substance misused in these samples.[11] Similarly, research sug-gests cannabis use is prevalent among young people at CHR-p, with 33% to 54% of youth at CHR-p using cannabis.[12] Although prevalence estimates vary across sam-ples, it is clear that cannabis use is common.

There are many reasons why adolescents who experience early psychosis may use cannabis. For one, adolescents who experience psychosis are influenced by similar considerations and pressures that may result in cannabis use for any adolescent. Cannabis use is increasingly common in adolescents (see Kristie Ladegard and Devika Bhatia's article, "Impact of Cannabis Legalization on Adolescent Cannabis Use," for review of cannabis use in adolescents). Trying new things (particularly things that

Table 1
Clinical high risk for psychosis versus first-episode psychosis case examples

CHR-p: David is a 14-year-old biracial (White-Southeast Asian) cis-male middle school student. David has started having difficulty paying attention in class and has had a drop in grades this past semester. David hears a voice he calls "Bada" about once a day that has been bothering him, but he always knows that this voice is his mind playing tricks on him. David has also started having the thought that his family has been replaced by actors; he notices this thought about once a week and he is always able to question it, but it makes him very uncomfortable and he may stay away from his family until the thought is gone. Because David can still doubt his experiences ("insight" intact), he could be described as exhibiting "attenuated" psychosis or CHR-p.

FEP: Sara is a 20-year-old Black trans-female college student studying economics. Sara started having the feeling that she was on earth for an important purpose but could not articulate it exactly. She started noticing hidden patterns and meanings in her economics textbooks and at school, which gave her information on the secrets to the universe. She stopped going to class to focus on these thoughts. She began mentioning these thoughts to her parents and roommate, and she dismissed their concerns that there may be something wrong and got angry when they suggested these thoughts may be incorrect. Her parents were worried and took her to the emergency room. Because Sara lost the ability to question her experiences and fully believed them (loss of "insight"), she could be described as experiencing acute psychosis or FEP.

young people observe in their peers) is common, suggesting that trying cannabis may be developmentally normative for youth. Substance use may also be one means for enhancing mood and promoting social ambition,[13] including goals of building social relationships and being perceived well by peers.

Some reasons for cannabis use may also be more specific to the experience of developing early psychosis. Research suggests that youth at CHR-p may use cannabis to alleviate some difficulties such as depression, anxiety, and negative symptoms, which commonly co-occur with or precede the onset of subthreshold (or attenuated) positive symptoms.[12] The "self-medication" hypothesis poses that young people may use cannabis because of a predisposition to psychosis, and individuals who are prone to psychosis may have a neurobiological predisposition to both cannabis use and psychotic illness.[12] After the onset of positive or other symptoms, substance use may be experienced as a way of coping with symptoms.[14] Overall, cannabis use is prevalent among young people experiencing early psychosis, and there are many reasons why this population uses it.

CLINICAL CONSIDERATIONS FOR OVERLAPPING PSYCHOSIS AND CANNABIS USE: DISCUSSION

Cannabis use has been associated with psychosis spectrum symptoms in several ways. First, in terms of incidence, research generally supports that there is a higher incidence of psychosis symptoms in people who use cannabis. In one study, the incidence of psychosis symptoms in adolescent cannabis users was 31%, compared with incidence of 20% in non–cannabis users.[15] Similarly, a systematic review described that most studies have indicated that cannabis consumption may lead to psychotic symptoms.[16] The Diagnostic and Statistical Manual (DSM) also includes a diagnosis of cannabis-induced psychotic disorder, in which people experience impairing psychotic symptoms that are directly caused by cannabis and not attributable to another (eg, underlying psychotic) disorder.

Several factors may increase the risk of experiencing psychosis for youth who use cannabis. Younger age of initiating cannabis use appears to be associated with increased risk of developing psychosis.[17] Cannabis strain is also important, with evidence that higher levels of THC compared with cannabidiol (CBD) are associated with greater risk for psychosis.[18] Concurrently, there is evidence that youth with FEP may preferentially use high potency cannabis (estimated 12%–18% THC).[19] In terms of method of administration, research suggests that inhalation of cannabis was associated with psychotic experiences in both adolescent and adults, although adults may be more vulnerable to acute psychotic symptoms than adolescents.[20] Some research suggests that people with psychosis who use cannabis are more likely to orally ingest oils, drinks, and tinctures and use topical forms of cannabis compared with controls.[21] Vaporized cannabis (vaping) is another common form of cannabis administration that has been found to induce stronger drug effects compared with smoked cannabis in adults, including higher paranoia ratings and cognitive impairment.[22] However, there does not seem to be comprehensive research directly comparing psychosis risk across methods of administration, but some methods may be prone to be higher potency. Overall, many factors influence the relationship between risk for developing psychosis and cannabis use, but there is a clear dose dependence such that earlier age of use and higher usage of THC-heavy cannabis is associated with poorer outcomes including psychosis.[23]

Consistent with adult schizophrenia research that persistent cannabis use is associated with negative outcomes (eg, worst psychotic symptoms, poorer functioning, decreased pleasure),[24,25] cannabis use is associated with negative outcomes for young people experiencing early psychosis. The vulnerability model asserts that individuals who are vulnerable to psychotic disorders have a "sensitive brain" that is susceptible to stressors like substances. Sensitivity to substances may result in an increase or exacerbation of psychosis symptoms.[14] Substance use in FEP has been associated with more hospitalizations, reduced treatment adherence, higher relapse rates, and higher cost of treatment.[12] Among several investigated substances, cannabis-induced psychosis was related to the highest conversion rate to acute psychosis.[26] In a meta-analysis, compared with nonusers, the heaviest cannabis users had a 4 times higher risk, and the average cannabis users had a 2 times higher risk for developing psychotic spectrum symptoms or disorders.[27] Concurrently, also consistent with adult schizophrenia research,[25] discontinuing cannabis use can improve symptoms for early psychosis. In FEP, reducing and stopping cannabis use is associated with improvements in psychotic symptoms,[28,29] and people with FEP who stop substance use have similar outcomes to people who had no prior substance use history.[29,30]

Despite generally negative associations with prognosis, there are complexities in research on how cannabis use may affect psychosis course for young people. In a study of how lifetime cannabis use contributed to psychosis outcomes in a CHR-p sample, low to moderate cannabis use did not contribute to conversion rate and was not associated with social and role functioning difficulties.[31] In addition, Bruins and colleagues (2021) found that cannabis use in a psychosis sample predicted worse psychosocial functioning and lower quality of life at baseline compared with nonusers, but after 1year found no significant differences between cannabis users and nonusers in psychosocial functioning or quality of life.[32] Some studies have found minimal cognitive deficits result from cannabis use in psychosis samples,[33,34] whereas other studies have found cannabis use is associated with poor cognitive outcomes in psychosis samples.[35]

Adding consideration of other diagnoses generally suggests heightened risks in other clinical groups. For example, people with borderline personality disorder who have a comorbid substance use disorder seem to experience increased psychotic symptoms from cannabis use.[36] Schizotypal personality disorder is also associated with a dose-response relationship between cannabis use and symptoms.[37] In addition, posttraumatic stress disorder is associated with increased psychosis symptoms resulting from cannabis use, particularly increased hallucinations.[38] In addition, childhood trauma and cannabis use seem to interact synergistically to heighten the risk of psychosis later in life.[39] However, perhaps surprisingly, research has not found that cannabis use is a significant risk factor for self-harm or suicide risk among people with psychosis[40,41] (but see Karla Molinero and Jesse D. Hinckley's article, "Adolescent Cannabis Use, Comorbid ADHD, and Other Internalizing and Externalizing Disorders," in this issue for more thorough review of mental health concerns associated with cannabis use).

Understanding the clinical overlap between cannabis and psychosis symptoms is an important piece of diagnostic conceptualization and treatment. However, the relationship between cannabis use and psychosis is complex. The current literature involves some conflicting findings and incomplete information. A great deal of existing research uses small sample sizes and is correlational, which results in uncertainty about confounds and direction of causality. Research is unclear whether cannabis itself causes psychosis, or if an underlying vulnerability to psychosis is triggered by cannabis use, or if people have an underlying vulnerability to cannabis *and* to psychosis. Overall, cannabis use likely represents a risk factor for onset and/or worsening of psychosis spectrum and other symptoms (see Section 7 for treatment considerations).

NEUROBIOLOGY OF OVERLAPPING PSYCHOSIS AND CANNABIS USE

Cannabis and psychosis have a complicated neurobiological overlap (see J. Cobb Scott's article, "Impact of Adolescent Cannabis Use on Neurocognitive and Brain Development," in this issue for a more comprehensive review). Some research has investigated differences in brain regions for young people with psychosis and cannabis use. Reduced gray matter density is a prominent feature of psychosis.[42] Adolescents with psychosis who use cannabis have reduced gray matter density compared with nonusers, suggesting that the brains of adolescents with psychosis may be particularly more vulnerable to the effects of cannabis.[42] FEP samples exposed to THC have decreased activity in the dorsolateral prefrontal cortex.[43] Bilateral thalamic volume loss[43] and right anterior hippocampal reduction[44] are also evident in cannabis users that have a family history of psychosis.

There is also consideration of how cannabis and psychosis may influence neurobiological functioning. In terms of brain activity, cannabis use is associated with lower resting global and prefrontal blood flow compared with nonusers with schizophrenia,[45] and THC exposure is associated with altered prefrontal cortex synaptic density and efficiency.[46] There is also evidence that thalamic hyperconnectivity with the sensory motor cortex seems to be associated with younger age of onset of cannabis use in clinical high risk for psychosisCHR-p.[47]

There is also research investigating how overlapping cannabis use and psychosis may be associated with changes at a neurotransmitter and receptor level in the brain. The endocannabinoid system is an important part of the central and peripheral nervous system that is affected by cannabis. Research suggests that the glutamatergic cognitive symptoms found in schizophrenia disorders might be a result of faults in the endocannabinoid system.[48] The CB1 receptor has been a focus because THC can be a CB1 agonist and contribute to the psychotomimetic effects of cannabis,[49] and CB1 may be associated with psychosis risk.[50] THC acts on the dopamine system as an agonist, increasing striatal and mesocorticolimbic dopamine levels. There seems to be a dose-response relationship between THC and its psychoactive effects.[51] Its impact on the dopamine system directly affects motor functioning, cognition, and emotional processing.[52] Although dopamine has been suggested as a possible factor in the cannabis-psychosis overlap, there is conflicting evidence of this relationship, including a systematic review that found that cannabis exposure may have a more tenuous than expected relationship with changes in the dopamine systems.[50] Finally, CBD is a component of cannabis that blocks the psychotogenic effects of THC.[53]

Overall, neurobiological research has identified ways in which cannabis may affect brain structures, connectivity, and neurotransmitter systems. Findings also suggest that people with psychosis and people with a family history of psychosis have altered brain structures that are further affected by cannabis use.

ASSESSMENT CONSIDERATIONS FOR PSYCHOSIS AND CANNABIS USE

The association between cannabis use and psychosis involves complexities and uncertainties in general and for particular clients. As a result, it is important to gather information about the timeline of both to inform diagnostic conceptualization and treatment recommendations. A timeline is necessary to consider relevant differential diagnoses, including cannabis-induced psychosis, which would require a client to have psychotic symptoms only following cannabis use. Assessment is important for building a shared understanding of experiences and clinical course over time, including onset, worsening, and relationship with patterns of behavior. It can be helpful to gather information from multiple sources (interview, collateral, self-report).

Several existing substance use assessments may be incorporated into clinical screening protocols, to increase the likelihood that clinical teams ask about use (see Jessica B Calihan and Sharon Levy's article, "Substance Use Screening, Brief Intervention, and Referral to Treatment in Pediatric Primary Care, School-based Health Clinics & Mental Health Clinics," in this issue). Self-report measures include the Brief Screener for Tobacco, Alcohol, and Other Drugs,[54] the Alcohol Expectancy Questionnaire-Brief,[55] and the Marijuana Effect Expectancy Questionnaire-Brief.[56] Existing early psychosis assessment tools include the Structured Interview for Psychosis-Risk Syndromes (SIPS),[57] which is a clinician-administered semistructured interview that gathers information relevant to whether a young person meets criteria for CHR-p and rates the severity of positive, negative, general, and disorganization symptoms. The SIPS involves building a timeline of psychosis spectrum and co-occurring concerns, which may include cannabis use.

Although these tools are useful for information gathering, providers often must accept some level of diagnostic uncertainty when seeing youth with these co-occurring concerns. See **Table 2** for case examples of how cannabis use and psychosis presentation might overlap.

TREATMENT CONSIDERATIONS FOR OVERLAPPING PSYCHOSIS AND CANNABIS USE

Because many people with psychosis also struggle with cannabis use and/or misuse, providers are commonly encouraged to target both clinical concerns in treatment. However, treatment may be fragmented for people who have dual diagnoses, as many separate treatment services for psychosis and substance use exist.[58] Psychosis

---

Table 2
Early psychosis-cannabis overlap case examples

Case 1: Rowan is a 19-year-old nonbinary Hispanic college student. They started noticing whispers and seeing shadows out of the corner of their eyes at age 16 y, which occurred about weekly and were mildly distracting but easy to ignore. They began trying cannabis with new college friends about once per week at age 18 y. They have noticed an increase in their perceptual changes since they started using cannabis, now daily and lasting a bit longer. About 3 months ago they also started noticing a distressing feeling that they are being watched by an evil force, about weekly, although they know this is likely their mind playing tricks on them. This timeline suggests that Rowan exhibited some risk for psychosis that has been exacerbated by cannabis use.

Case 2: Sam is a 24-year-old White cis-female administrator. She has long-standing difficulties with social anxiety and over the last 2 y has been using more cannabis to help her sleep, nightly. About 6 months ago, she began to experience increased suspiciousness (concerns about surveillance, checking for cameras) and thoughts that she must figure out a "game" that has been created for her. These thoughts became compelling and led her to withdraw from some daily activities, but she is not fully sure about the game. This timeline suggests that Sam's psychosis symptoms may stem from cannabis use, but it remains unclear from this information whether she has underlying psychosis vulnerability or whether these symptoms would persist if she stopped use.

and substance use may be exclusions for specialized treatment programs (eg, FEP programs may exclude young people with clear substance–induced psychosis). Because clinicians are often tasked with providing treatment to young people with both concerns, providers are encouraged to learn about managing co-occurring symptoms. This section provides an overview (and see Jessica B Calihan and Sharon Levy's article, "Substance Use Screening, Brief Intervention, and Referral to Treatment in Pediatric Primary Care, School-based Health Clinics & Mental Health Clinics," in this issue and Winters and colleagues' article, "Brief Interventions for Cannabis Using Adolescents," in this issue), **Table 3** refers to additional informational resources, and **Table 4** highlights key clinical guidelines and strategies.

Based on research that cannabis use is associated with risk for worsening psychosis (see Section 4), reducing or abstaining from cannabis use is a common treatment emphasis for youth with these co-occurring concerns. Youth who present with acute psychosis in the context of cannabis use are commonly advised to discontinue use and prescribed antipsychotics.[58] Antipsychotics (eg, risperidone) have been used to treat dual diagnosis of substance use disorders and psychosis in adults.[59] Offering psychoeducation and antipsychotics early in the course of psychosis may reduce both current positive psychotic symptoms and substance use and may prevent future episodes of substance use and untreated psychosis.[58] For ongoing treatment, treatment teams including a therapist, psychiatrist, and the family are most effective in treating dual diagnosis of psychosis and substance use in adults.[60] Similarly, increasing research supports the effectiveness of specialized team–based treatment programs for young people with early psychosis (both FEP and CHR-p), called "coordinated specialty care."[61] Programs that focus on engagement of family, psychoeducation, individual and group therapy, and the lowest effective dose of medications prove best outcomes for early psychosis populations.[58] These multidisciplinary treatment teams typically treat psychosis and substance use, guided by treatment strategies for substance use disorders in adults. Work examining treatment practices for dual diagnosis of psychosis and substance use in young people suggests that clients should first be offered generalized early psychosis interventions, and specialist substance use programs should be offered to clients who do not improve from early psychosis treatment alone.[62]

Table 3 Early psychosis resources	
Organization	**Website**
PEPPNET Webinars/Conferences	https://med.stanford.edu/peppnet
EPICENTER Speaker Series	https://medicine.osu.edu/departments/psychiatry-and-behavioral-health/epicenter/epicenter-speaker-series
National Association of State Mental Health Program Directors	https://www.nasmhpd.org/webinars
SAMHSA/CMHS: Substance-Induced Psychosis in First Episode Programming	https://www.nasmhpd.org/sites/default/files/DH-Substance-Induced-Psychosisin-First-Episode-Programming%20_0.pdf
SAMHSA/CMHS: Treating Affective Psychosis and Substance Use Disorders Within Coordinated Specialty Care	https://www.nasmhpd.org/sites/default/files/DH-TreatingAffectivePsychosis_v2.pdf
SAMHSA/CMHS: Cognitive Behavioral Therapy for Psychosis (CBTp)	https://www.nasmhpd.org/sites/default/files/DH-CBTp_Fact_Sheet.pdf

Table 4 Clinic care points	
Client Care Main Points	• Treatment engagement is key • Emphasize client interests and life goals • Assess both psychosis and cannabis use (at intake and throughout treatment) • Give feedback that cannabis use risks increasing psychotic symptoms • Start by offering clients generalized early psychosis treatment • Substance use interventions that may be incorporated into treatment include motivational interviewing (MI) and harm reduction • Family treatment may be effective at reducing use • Specialist substance use treatment should be offered to clients who do not improve from early psychosis treatment alone
Strategies for Asking About Cannabis Use	• Do you know people or have friends who have tried weed/ pot/marijuana? • How often do you use weed/pot/marijuana? • Do you remember what first made you curious to try weed/ pot/marijuana? • When do you like using weed? • What do you like about using it? • Is there anything that bothers you about using weed? (ask about likes first) • Are you curious to hear how weed may affect psychosis symptoms like? (add examples as relevant to the client)
Therapy Strategies for Cannabis Use	• Gather information about what the client likes/dislikes about using and what situations typically lead client to use (eg, boredom, enjoyment with peers, reduced anxiety, improved sleep) • Adapt to client's stage of change • Gather information about times the client has thought about or tried to cut back • Identify concerns and barriers to reducing cannabis use (eg, peers using) • Reinforce curiosity (eg, "some people find that reducing weed use decreases their hallucinations, I'm curious whether that would be true for you too?"), send information, encourage client to read or look up information to discuss in treatment • Develop a specific plan for reduced use together (when, how long) • Create barriers to using (eg, ask friends/family to call you out for using or resist sharing cannabis with you) • Cope ahead for expected difficulties (eg, urges to use, responses to peers who offer cannabis, find alternate activities for times when you would typically use)

Core treatment priorities for co-occurring psychosis and cannabis use include assessing both symptoms, prioritizing engagement in treatment, and highlighting risks of cannabis use in a clinically appropriate way. Maintaining treatment engagement increases the likelihood that young people will share details about their experience of cannabis use. In terms of clinical style, providers are encouraged to maintain open curiosity, normalize reasons for use, and refrain from lecturing. At the same time, providers can note that there is evidence that cannabis can increase risk of new or worsening psychosis symptoms (see Section 4) and can encourage young people to consider the overlap in their treatment.

Specific substance use interventions that may be incorporated into treatment include motivational interviewing, cognitive behavioral therapy, and a focus on interests and life goals.[62] Motivational interviewing involves using an attitude of benevolent curiosity to gather the client's observations about their cannabis use and what they like and dislike about cannabis and adjusting to the client's "stage of change." It can include sharing information about how cannabis and psychosis symptoms may affect each other, reinforcing any client concerns about negative impacts of use, enhancing any client-expressed curiosity about reducing cannabis use, strategizing with clients who express interest in reducing use (eg, ask for help from friends, arrange for drug testing), and trying breaks from cannabis use as an "experiment." Harm reduction involves identifying ways to reduce cannabis use (without necessarily aiming for abstinence) and may include strategies such as using cannabis with lower THC, reducing frequency of use during the day, pausing during episodes of use, and planning use in safer contexts. Finally, families are commonly included in early psychosis treatment.[63] There is some research on training parents with motivational interviewing strategies, both for early psychosis symptoms and for cannabis cravings and use.[64,65] Although these strategies are commonly taught and incorporated informally into standard early psychosis treatment, these is less research formally assessing their effectiveness in early psychosis samples.

GAPS IN RESEARCH AND FUTURE DIRECTIONS

Although research has generally suggested that cannabis use may contribute to development of psychosis symptoms and likely negatively affects course of psychosis risk and psychotic disorders in young people, the overlap between psychosis and cannabis is not fully understood. A great deal of existing research on the overlap uses small sample sizes and is correlational, so larger scale, longitudinal research decrease uncertainty about confounds and direction of causality. There are gaps in understanding the complicated clinical and neurobiological picture in psychosis risk (CHR-p) and cannabis use; it seems a subset of clients at CHR-p continue to use cannabis at some level without experiencing conversion to acute psychosis. Although there are some factors that seem to contribute to risk of conversion (eg, early use, higher potency use), it is unclear what other variables may make some youth more likely to develop acute psychosis. There are also some mixed findings about negative outcomes for young people with co-occurring psychosis and cannabis use (eg, functioning, cognition).

Despite available guidelines (see Section 7), there is limited systematic treatment research (eg, randomized controlled trials) establishing effective evidence-based care for co-occurring early psychosis and cannabis use. Although preliminary work suggests that early psychosis treatments are effective at treating both, more research is needed about the effectiveness of specific strategies (motivational interviewing, harm reduction). In addition, there is limited research investigating which antipsychotic medications to prescribe for psychotic symptoms that seem caused or worsened by cannabis or at what point to start them (eg, based on severity of attenuated symptoms?). Future research also seems to be considering nonantipsychotic treatments for co-occurring psychosis and cannabis use. For example, some researchers have explored whether CBD may be an effective treatment of reduction of psychosis symptoms, including one study finding that CBD was associated with reductions in positive symptoms for participants with schizophrenia[66] and another finding that CBD improved brain functioning in participants at CHR-p.[67] Although these preliminary results suggest clinical utility, CBD interventions require further research (including randomized controlled trials) to inform the best evidence-based care.[68]

SUMMARY

Overall, psychosis and cannabis use may overlap in multiple ways in young people. Research suggests that cannabis use increases risk for having psychotic symptoms, both attenuated (subthreshold) and acute. Cannabis use may also exacerbate psychosis symptoms among young people with underlying psychosis risk and psychotic disorders. Although there are suggestions for treating co-occurring psychosis and cannabis use in young people (eg, incorporating cannabis use assessment and treatment strategies into specialized early psychosis care), there are many gaps in clinical trial research to support evidence-based treatment of these overlapping concerns.

DISCLOSURE

The authors report no disclosures or conflicts of interest.

ACKNOWLEDGMENTS

The authors would like to thank the following groups, institutions, and individuals for their support: University of Colorado School of Medicine (CUSOM) Department of Psychiatry (DoP); DoP Adult Division; DoP Division of Addiction Science, Prevention, and Treatment; Program for Early Assessment, Care, and Study (PEACS) team and trainees including Melissa Batt, MD, Charles Buteyn, LCSW, Christine Reed, MA, Madison Barber, Shanna Trott; mentors of the co-authors including Laura Anthony, PhD, Michelle-Friedman-Yakoobian, PhD, Shirley Yen, PhD, and William Stone, PhD; and volume editors Jessica Megan Ross, PhD, Paula Riggs, MD, and Jesse D Hinckley, MD.

REFERENCES

1. Fusar-Poli P, Papanastasiou E, Stahl D, et al. Treatments of negative symptoms in schizophrenia: meta-analysis of 168 randomized placebo-controlled trials. Schizophr Bull 2015;41(4):892–9.
2. Remschmidt H. Early-onset schizophrenia as a progressive-deteriorating developmental disorder: evidence from child psychiatry. J Neural Transm (Vienna) 2002;109(1):101–17.
3. Coulon N, Godin O, Bulzacka E, et al. Early and very early-onset schizophrenia compared with adult-onset schizophrenia: French FACE-SZ database. Brain Behav 2020;10(2):e01495.
4. Addington J, Liu L, Buchy L, et al. North american prodrome longitudinal study (NAPLS 2): the prodromal symptoms. J Nerv Ment Dis 2015;203(5):328–35.
5. Fusar-Poli P, Bechdolf A, Taylor MJ, et al. At risk for schizophrenic or affective psychoses? A meta-analysis of DSM/ICD diagnostic outcomes in individuals at high clinical risk. Schizophr Bull 2013;39(4):923–32.
6. Agius M, Zaman R, Hanafy D. An audit to assess the consequences of the use of a pluripotential risk syndrome: the case to move on from "psychosis risk syndrome (PRS). Psychiatr Danub 2013;25(Suppl 2):S282–5.

7. Simon GE, Coleman KJ, Yarborough BJH, et al. First Presentation with psychotic symptoms in a population-based sample. Psychiatr Serv 2017;68(5):456–61.
8. Kidd SA, Howison M, Pilling M, et al. Severe mental illness in LGBT populations: a scoping review. Psychiatr Serv 2016;67(7):779–83, published correction appears in psychiatr serv. 2016 May 1;67(5):550.
9. Scandurra C, Mezza F, Maldonato NM, et al. Health of non-binary and genderqueer people: a systematic review. Front Psychol 2019;10:1453–2019.
10. Yung AR, Nelson B, Baker K, et al. Psychotic-like experiences in a community sample of adolescents: implications for the continuum model of psychosis and prediction of schizophrenia. Aust N Z J Psychiatry 2009;43(2):118–28.
11. Batalla A, Garcia-Rizo C, Castellví P, et al. Screening for substance use disorders in first-episode psychosis: implications for readmission. Schizophr Res 2013; 146(1–3):125–31.
12. Addington J, Case N, Saleem MM, et al. Substance use in clinical high risk for psychosis: a review of the literature. Early Interv Psychiatry 2014;8(2):104–12.
13. Gill KE, Poe L, Azimov N, et al. Reasons for cannabis use among youths at ultra high risk for psychosis. Early Interv Psychiatry 2015;9(3):207–10.
14. Addington J, Addington D. Impact of an early psychosis program on substance use. Psychiatr Rehabil J 2001;25(1):60–7.
15. Kuepper R, van Os J, Lieb R, et al. Continued cannabis use and risk of incidence and persistence of psychotic symptoms: 10 year follow-up cohort study. BMJ 2011;342:d738.
16. Ortiz-Medina MB, Perea M, Torales J, et al. Cannabis consumption and psychosis or schizophrenia development. Int J Soc Psychiatry 2018;64(7):690–704.
17. Chadwick B, Miller ML, Hurd YL. Cannabis use during adolescent development: susceptibility to psychiatric illness. Front Psychiatry 2013;4:129.
18. Englund A, Morrison PD, Nottage J, et al. Cannabidiol inhibits THC-elicited paranoid symptoms and hippocampal-dependent memory impairment. J Psychopharmacol 2013;27(1):19–27.
19. Di Forti M, Morgan C, Dazzan P, et al. High-potency cannabis and the risk of psychosis. Br J Psychiatry 2009;195(6):488–91.
20. Mokrysz C, Shaban NDC, Freeman TP, et al. Acute effects of cannabis on speech illusions and psychotic-like symptoms: two studies testing the moderating effects of cannabidiol and adolescence. Psychol Med 2020;1–9. https://doi.org/10.1017/S0033291720001038.
21. Rup J, Freeman TP, Perlman C, et al. Cannabis and mental health: prevalence of use and modes of cannabis administration by mental health status. Addict Behav 2021;121:106991.
22. Spindle TR, Cone EJ, Schlienz NJ, et al. Acute effects of smoked and vaporized cannabis in healthy adults who infrequently use cannabis: a crossover trial. JAMA Netw Open 2018;1(7):e184841, published correction appears in JAMA Netw Open. 2018 Dec 7;1(8):e187241.
23. Bagot KS, Milin R, Kaminer Y. Adolescent initiation of cannabis use and early-onset psychosis. Subst Abus 2015;36(4):524–33.
24. Schnakenberg Martin AM, Lysaker PH. Individuals with psychosis and a lifetime history of cannabis use show greater deficits in emotional experience compared to non-using peers. J Ment Health 2020;29(1):77–83.
25. Setién-Suero E, Neergaard K, Ortiz-García de la Foz V, et al. Stopping cannabis use benefits outcome in psychosis: findings from 10-year follow-up study in the PAFIP-cohort. Acta Psychiatr Scand 2019;140(4):349–59.

26. Niemi-Pynttäri JA, Sund R, Putkonen H, et al. Substance-induced psychoses converting into schizophrenia: a register-based study of 18,478 Finnish inpatient cases. J Clin Psychiatry 2013;74(1):e94–9.
27. Marconi A, Di Forti M, Lewis CM, et al. Meta-analysis of the association between the level of cannabis use and risk of psychosis. Schizophr Bull 2016;42(5): 1262–9.
28. González-Pinto A, Alberich S, Barbeito S, et al. Cannabis and first-episode psychosis: different long-term outcomes depending on continued or discontinued use. Schizophr Bull 2011;37(3):631–9.
29. Mullin K, Gupta P, Compton MT, et al. Large M. Does giving up substance use work for patients with psychosis? A systematic meta-analysis. Aust NZJ Psychiatry 2012;46(9):826–39.
30. Weibell MA, Hegelstad WTV, Auestad B, et al. The effect of substance use on 10-year outcome in first-episode psychosis. Schizophr Bull 2017;43(4):843–51.
31. Auther AM, McLaughlin D, Carrión RE, et al. Prospective study of cannabis use in adolescents at clinical high risk for psychosis: impact on conversion to psychosis and functional outcome. Psychol Med 2012;42(12):2485–97.
32. Bruins J, Pijnenborg GHM, PHAMOUS investigators, et al. The association of cannabis use with quality of life and psychosocial functioning in psychosis. Schizophr Res 2021;228:229–34.
33. Scott JC, Slomiak ST, Jones JD, et al. Association of cannabis with cognitive functioning in adolescents and young adults: a systematic review and meta-analysis. JAMA Psychiatry 2018;75(6):585–95.
34. de Vos C, Leopold K, Blanke ES, et al. The relationship between cannabis use and cognition in people diagnosed with first-episode psychosis. Psychiatry Res 2020;293:113424.
35. Levine A, Clemenza K, Rynn M, et al. Evidence for the risks and consequences of adolescent cannabis exposure. J Am Acad Child Adolesc Psychiatry 2017;56(3): 214–25.
36. Barral C, Rodríguez-Cintas L, Grau-López L, et al. Substance-induced psychotic symptoms in Borderline Personality Disorder among substance use disorder samples in Spain. Psychiatry Res 2018;260:313–7.
37. Davis GP, Compton MT, Wang S, et al. Association between cannabis use, psychosis, and schizotypal personality disorder: findings from the National Epidemiologic Survey on Alcohol and Related Conditions. Schizophr Res 2013;151(1–3): 197–202.
38. Auxéméry Y, Fidelle G. Psychose. Et traumatisme psychique. Pour une articulation théorique des symptômes psycho-traumatiques et psychotiques chroniques [Psychosis and trauma. Theorical links between post-traumatic and psychotic symptoms]. Encephale 2011;37(6):433–8.
39. Khokhar JY, Dwiel LL, Henricks AM, et al. The link between schizophrenia and substance use disorder: a unifying hypothesis. Schizophr Res 2018;194:78–85.
40. Uliana V, Tomassini A, Pollice R, et al. Cannabis and psychosis: a systematic review of genetic studies. Curr Psychiatry Rev 2013;9:302–15.
41. Large M, Mullin K, Gupta P, et al. Systematic meta-analysis of outcomes associated with psychosis and co-morbid substance use. Aust N Z J Psychiatry 2014; 48(5):418–32.
42. Abush H, Ghose S, Van Enkevort EA, et al. Associations between adolescent cannabis use and brain structure in psychosis. Psychiatry Res Neuroimaging 2018;276:53–64.

43. Cupo L, Plitman E, Guma E, et al. A systematic review of neuroimaging and acute cannabis exposure in age-of-risk for psychosis. Transl Psychiatry 2021;11(1):217.

44. Welch KA, Stanfield AC, McIntosh AM, et al. Impact of cannabis use on thalamic volume in people at familial high risk of schizophrenia. Br J Psychiatry 2011; 199(5):386–90.

45. Jockers-Scherübl MC, Rentzsch J, Danker-Hopfe H, et al. Adequate antipsychotic treatment normalizes serum nerve growth factor concentrations in schizophrenia with and without cannabis or additional substance abuse. Neurosci Lett 2006;400(3):262–6.

46. D'Souza DC, Sewell RA, Ranganathan M. Cannabis and psychosis/schizophrenia: human studies. Eur Arch Psychiatry Clin Neurosci 2009;259(7):413–31.

47. Buchy L, Cannon TD, Anticevic A, et al. Evaluating the impact of cannabis use on thalamic connectivity in youth at clinical high risk of psychosis. BMC Psychiatry 2015;15:276.

48. Vigano D, Guidali C, Petrosino S, et al. Involvement of the endocannabinoid system in phencyclidine-induced cognitive deficits modelling schizophrenia. Int J Neuropsychopharmacol 2009;12(5):599–614.

49. Pertwee RG. The diverse CB1 and CB2 receptor pharmacology of three plant cannabinoids: delta9-tetrahydrocannabinol, cannabidiol and delta9-tetrahydrocannabivarin. Br J Pharmacol 2008;153(2):199–215.

50. Sami MB, Bhattacharyya S. Are cannabis-using and non-using patients different groups? Towards understanding the neurobiology of cannabis use in psychotic disorders. J Psychopharmacol 2018;32(8):825–49.

51. Shrivastava A, Johnston M, Terpstra K, et al. Cannabis and psychosis: neurobiology. Indian J Psychiatry 2014;56(1):8–16.

52. Delisi LE, Bertisch HC, Szulc KU, et al. A preliminary DTI study showing no brain structural change associated with adolescent cannabis use. Harm Reduct J 2006;3:17.

53. Bhattacharyya S, Morrison PD, Fusar-Poli P, et al. Opposite effects of delta-9-tetrahydrocannabinol and cannabidiol on human brain function and psychopathology. Neuropsychopharmacology 2010;35(3):764–74.

54. Kelly SM, Gryczynski J, Mitchell SG, et al. Validity of brief screening instrument for adolescent tobacco, alcohol, and drug use. Pediatrics 2014;133(5):819–26.

55. Stein LA, Katz B, Colby SM, et al. Validity and reliability of the alcohol expectancy questionnaire-adolescent, brief. J Child Adolesc Subst Abuse 2007;16(2): 115–27.

56. Torrealday O, Stein LA, Barnett N, et al. Validation of the marijuana effect expectancy questionnaire-brief. J Child Adolesc Subst Abuse 2008;17(4):1–17.

57. McGlashan TH, Walsh BC, Woods SW. The psychosis-risk syndrome: handbook for diagnosis and follow-up. New York: Oxford University Press; 2010.

58. Goerke D, Kumra S. Substance abuse and psychosis. Child Adolesc Psychiatr Clin N Am 2013;22(4):643–54.

59. Temmingh HS, Williams T, Siegfried N, et al. Risperidone versus other antipsychotics for people with severe mental illness and co-occurring substance misuse. Cochrane Database Syst Rev 2018;1(1):CD011057.

60. Barrowclough C, Haddock G, Tarrier N, et al. Randomized controlled trial of motivational interviewing, cognitive behavior therapy, and family intervention for patients with comorbid schizophrenia and substance use disorders. Am J Psychiatry 2001;158(10):1706–13.

61. Sherrill J, Goldstein AB, Azrin ST. Evidence-based treatments for first episode psychosis: components of coordinated specialty care. Bethesda, MD: NIMH; 2014.
62. Substance Abuse and Mental Health Services Administration. First-Episode Psychosis and Co-Occurring Substance Use Disorders. Rockville, MD: National Mental Health and Substance Use Policy Laboratory; 2019.
63. Gupta M, Bowie CR. Family cohesion and flexibility in early episode psychosis. Early Interv Psychiatry 2018;12(5):886–92.
64. Kline ER, Thibeau H, Sanders AS, et al. Motivational interviewing for loved ones in early psychosis: development and pilot feasibility trial of a brief psychoeducational intervention for caregivers. Front Psychiatry 2021;12:659568.
65. Smeerdijk M, Keet R, Dekker N, et al. Motivational interviewing and interaction skills training for parents to change cannabis use in young adults with recent-onset schizophrenia: a randomized controlled trial. Psychol Med 2012;42(8): 1627–36.
66. McGuire P, Robson P, Cubala WJ, et al. Cannabidiol (CBD) as an adjunctive therapy in schizophrenia: a multicenter randomized controlled trial. Am J Psychiatry 2018;175(3):225–31.
67. Bhattacharyya S, Wilson R, Appiah-Kusi E, et al. Effect of cannabidiol on medial temporal, midbrain, and striatal dysfunction in people at clinical high risk of psychosis: a randomized clinical trial. JAMA Psychiatry 2018;75(11):1107–17.
68. Hahn B. The potential of cannabidiol treatment for cannabis users with recent-onset psychosis. Schizophr Bull 2018;44(1):46–53.

A Review of the Effects of Adolescent Cannabis Use on Physical Health

Abigail L. Tuvel, BA[a], Evan A. Winiger, PhD[b], J. Megan Ross, PhD[c,*]

KEYWORDS

- Pulmonary • Cardiovascular • Gastrointestinal • Endocrine • Body mass index
- Sleep • Cannabis • Physical health

KEY POINTS

- Adolescents who vape are at risk for e-cigarette or vaping product use–associated lung injury.
- Various case studies support that adolescents who use cannabis can develop cannabinoid hyperemesis syndrome.
- Cannabis use is associated with a lower body mass index among adolescents.
- Research is inconclusive on the impact of cannabis use on heart rate and blood pressure.
- Cannabis use among adolescents is associated with various sleep outcomes such as insomnia, shorter sleep time, later bedtimes, and greater endorsement of sleep problems.

INTRODUCTION

Adolescence is a time marked by various physical, psychological, and social changes, typically including initiation of substance use such as cannabis.[1–3] Increasing evidence suggests that cannabis use is not harmless, especially during periods of critical development.[4–6] As laws change around recreational and medical use of cannabis, prevalence of use in certain populations has changed too. Overall, prevalence of adult cannabis use has increased, whereas prevalence of adolescent use has seemed to remain steady or even decrease.[4,7–10] However, most of the studies that examined the impact of recreational and medical cannabis legalization on adolescent cannabis

This article originally appeared in *Child and Adolescent Psychiatric Clinics*, Volume 32 Issue 1, January 2023.
[a] Department of Psychology and Neuroscience, University of Colorado Boulder, 1777 Exposition Drive, Boulder, CO 80301; [b] Department of Psychiatry, School of Medicine, University of Colorado Anschutz Medical Campus, 1890 N Revere Court, Aurora, CO, 80045; [c] Department of Psychiatry, Division of Addiction Sciences, Treatment and Prevention, University of Colorado Anschutz Medical Campus, 1890 N Revere Court, Aurora, CO, 80045
* Corresponding author.
E-mail address: Jessica.M.Ross@cuanschutz.edu

Psychiatr Clin N Am 46 (2023) 719–739
https://doi.org/10.1016/j.psc.2023.03.005
0193-953X/23/Published by Elsevier Inc.

use do not consider frequency of use and/or potency of products that may have increased among adolescents. Nonetheless, cannabis use is still widespread among adolescents, with greater than 10% of 8th graders and greater than 35% of 12th graders endorsing use in the past year.[10] The substantial portion of adolescents reporting cannabis use illuminates the need for further research into possible adverse health risks. Most of the research focused on this topic has been conducted with adults, with some newer adolescent studies emerging in the last decade.[11–14] This review outlines the current research on how cannabis use affects physical health in adolescence.

Smoking cannabis seems to be the most frequent method of use by adolescents, but vaping may be gaining popularity.[10,15] Results from the 2020 Monitoring the Future survey show that in eighth grade students there was a small increase in vaping cannabis. This trend was not observed in 10th and 12th grade students. However, in 2018 and 2019, increases in vaping both cannabis and nicotine were observed in all these age groups. Overall, 2020 rates for cannabis vaping annually were 8.1%, 19.1%, and 22.1%, for students in 8th, 10th, and 12th grade, respectively.[10] Other recent, large studies have found similar levels of cannabis vaping in adolescents.[16,17] Concentrates, or high-potency cannabis products, are also gaining popularity among adolescents, 72% of adolescents who endorse cannabis use report using concentrates at least once in their lifetime.[18]

After changes in medical and recreational cannabis legalization in various states across the United States, concerns around adolescents having greater access to cannabis has driven research into possible changes and differences in adolescent use in legal versus nonlegal states.[4,9,19–21] Most of the studies focused on adolescent cannabis use patterns in medically legal states have not found any significant differences in adolescent use prevalence compared to nonmedically legal states.[21–23] However, one study did observe an increase in first-time adolescent cannabis use in medically legal states but not a subsequent increase in regular use.[22] Another study did detect an increased rate of cannabis use in adolescents living in medically legal versus nonlegal states but highlighted that even before legalization, these now medically legal states had higher levels of adolescent use compared to non legal states.[24] Less research has been conducted on recreational cannabis legality and subsequent adolescent use, as these laws have been passed more recently, and there is little conclusive evidence to support any effect at this time.[9,19]

This review includes research about the associations between cannabis use and indicators of physical health. The authors include studies addressing the association between cannabis use and pulmonary, cardiovascular, gastrointestinal, and endocrine function, as well as body mass index (BMI) and sleep. **Table 1** provides an overview of clinical concerns for each of the body systems/constructs for adolescents who use cannabis. One major limitation of this research review is that most of this research has been conducted with adults rather than adolescents.

PULMONARY FUNCTION

The most common method of cannabis intake for adolescents is smoking.[15] Most research on the impact of cannabis use on pulmonary function has focused on comparing the effects of cannabis smoking to the effects of tobacco smoking, as tobacco smoking has known health risks that have been replicated in many studies.[25–30] Most of the existing literature on pulmonary function comes from adult studies.[12,27,31] These studies assess various aspects of pulmonary function, with an emphasis on respiratory symptoms, lung function, and pulmonary diseases and disorders.[12,27,31–33]

Table 1	
Physical health clinical concerns for adolescent who use cannabis	
System/ Construct	**Clinical Concern**
Pulmonary	• E-cigarette or vaping product use–associated lung injury (EVALI)
Cardiovascular	• Acute cardiovascular events (eg, myocardial infarction, atrial fibrillation, acute coronary syndromes [stroke], ventricular tachycardia, and sudden death)
Gastrointestinal	• Cannabinoid hyperemesis syndrome (CHS) • Nausea, stomach pain, and appetite loss during cannabis withdrawal
Endocrine	• Disruption of normal cortisol function throughout the day • Decreased stress reactivity
Body mass index (BMI)	• Lower BMI
Sleep	• Insomnia • Insufficient sleep on school nights • Shorter total sleep time • Later bedtimes • Evening chronotype

However, recent research is emerging on e-cigarette or vaping product use–associated lung injury (EVALI), with particular concern involving cases among adolescents and young adults.[34–36]

Research on cannabis use and respiratory symptoms has identified associations between smoking cannabis and coughing, wheezing, shortness of breath, and sputum production. Higher rates of coughing, sputum production, and wheezing in adults who use cannabis compared to those who do not have been found in several studies, even when controlling for tobacco use.[29,32,33,37] Rates of these symptoms in those who use cannabis were comparable with those who use tobacco, with some studies finding a higher prevalence of these symptoms in those who use cannabis compared to those who use tobacco or finding that cannabis and tobacco co-use resulted in higher rates of these symptoms.[29,32,33]

Existing literature on cannabis use and lung function relies on spirometry measures such as forced expiratory volume in 1 second (FEV1) and forced vital capacity (FVC). The ratio of FEV1 to FVC is used to measure lung function and progression of disease, especially chronic obstructive pulmonary disease (COPD), with lower ratios indicating more airflow obstruction.[38,39] Results from these studies have been inconclusive, with many reporting conflicting results for the effect of smoking cannabis on FEV1, FVC, and FEV1/FVC ratios.[12,26–29,32,40] For example, Aldington and colleagues[26] (2007) found a dose-response association between amount of cannabis exposure and lower FEV1/FVC ratios. In contrast, Hancox and colleagues[27] (2010) found cannabis exposure to be associated with higher FVC measurements, but was not found to be associated with FEV1/FVC ratios. Future studies are needed to settle the debate on whether cannabis smoking negatively affects lung function.

Attention has been given to the potential for cannabis use to increase risk for pulmonary diseases and disorders, such as asthma, COPD, lung cancer, and severe bronchitis. So far, studies on this topic have only been conducted with adults.[25,30,31,41,42] Newer research has shown support for an association between asthma and cannabis use, and a recent study reported that emerging adults who currently use cannabis had a 1.71 odds ratio for filling prescriptions for asthma, even after controlling for relevant covariates such as BMI and tobacco use.[30,31] Studies that support an association between cannabis use and COPD are limited, but there is compelling research evidence to support an increased risk for severe or chronic bronchitis in those who use cannabis.[30,42–44] Finally, early research on cannabis smoking and risk of lung cancer has found some support for a possible association but has not yielded any conclusive results yet.[25,40,41,43] However, a recent, large-scale, longitudinal study investigating this association has found that adults who chronically use cannabis had an increased risk for lung cancer, suggesting that at high levels, cannabis smoking may have serious long-term detrimental effects on the lungs.[41]

Of the possible pulmonary-related effects of adolescent cannabis use, perhaps the most immediately concerning is the incidence of EVALI. With greater than 15% of EVALI cases occurring in adolescents, and 37.2% of adolescents in the Monitoring the Future 2020 survey reporting vaping, this issue is critically important, even though cases are not as high as they were during the initial EVALI outbreak in 2019.[10,34–36] Thakrar and colleagues[36] (2020) conducted a review of 12 adolescent EVALI cases and found that 100% of the patients had confluent ground-glass opacities and 92% had centrilobular ground-glass nodules present in their chest computed tomography scans. Other commonly occurring pulmonary effects of EVALI include respiratory symptoms such as shortness of breath, pain in the chest, cough, and more rarely, hemoptysis.[45,46] The median age of individuals who died as a result of EVALI was 51 years old, but the youngest recorded was 15 years old.[47] Texas and Illinois have the highest number of EVALI cases, and nonregulated delta-9-tetrahydrocannabinol (THC)-containing vaping products are more likely to result in injury compared to products that do not contain THC.[34,45]

CARDIOVASCULAR FUNCTION

The impact of cannabis use on cardiovascular health is unclear because research has reported mixed results. Most research of cannabis use and cardiovascular function have focused on heart rate and blood pressure; thus this section focuses on those 2 outcomes as well. However, no studies have examined the impact of cannabis use on heart rate and blood pressure in a sample of adolescents.

Most research on the impact of cannabis use on heart rate has focused on acute effects. All research suggest that acute cannabis intoxication is associated with an increased heart rate.[48,49] Furthermore, one randomized controlled trial of cannabis use found that smoked cannabis was associated with an increased heart rate, and the feeling of being "high" was positively associated with heart rate. Heart rate peaked after 10 minutes of smoking cannabis and the increased heart rate went down to pre-use levels after 40 minutes.[49] Another study of acute cannabis intoxication found that after smoking cannabis, heart rate and salivary THC levels were positively associated.[48] However, both samples include less than 15 participants, so substantial conclusions about the association between heart rate and acute cannabis intoxication cannot be made. Although rare, a series of case reports have found that there are documented deaths of young adults from acute cardiovascular events after recently ingesting cannabis.[50] Although rare, myocardial infarction can occur within 60 minutes of ingesting cannabis.[51] Furthermore, other cardiovascular events have been found following cannabis ingestion including atrial fibrillation, acute coronary syndromes (such as stroke), ventricular tachycardia, and even sudden death. These effects were found in young patients without any other risk factors for cardiovascular events.[52] The long-term effects of cannabis use on heart rate are less clear. One study examined 72 men who tested positive for THC and 72 matched controls and found that heart rate variability was higher among those who tested positive for THC compared to controls.[53] However, a recent co-twin control study found that cannabis frequency was negatively associated with resting heart rate finding that more frequent cannabis use was associated with a lower resting heart rate.[54]

Acutely, cannabis use is associated with reduced blood pressure but this has only been documented in animal studies.[55] Long-term effects are also unclear. One study that included more than 12,000 adults reported a positive dose-dependent association between past 30-day cannabis use and systolic blood pressure. Each additional day of cannabis use was associated with increased 0.10 mmHG in systolic blood pressure; however, the clinical significance of this increase is unclear.[56] Two additional studies found that cannabis use, measured in joint-years, was associated with lower systolic and diastolic blood pressure among adults.[57,58] One co-twin control study did not find evidence of a causal association between cannabis frequency and systolic or diastolic blood pressure.[54] Finally, several studies have examined what happens to blood pressure during cannabis cessation, finding no significant change in blood pressure,[59] whereas one small crossover study found increases in blood pressure during cannabis cessation.[60]

GASTROINTESTINAL FUNCTION

The current research focused on cannabis use, and gastrointestinal function includes cannabinoid hyperemesis syndrome, cannabis withdrawal syndrome, and the medicinal use of cannabis for treating digestive disorders such as inflammatory bowel disease.[13,61–63] Most of these studies include only adults rather than adolescents or are limited by small sample sizes.[64–67] Few studies address specific cannabinoids (CBD) in their analyses on the effect of cannabis on gastrointestinal function. However, there is research about the potential for CBD to treat digestive disorder symptoms, but this research has yielded inconclusive findings.[68–70]

Cannabinoid hyperemesis syndrome (CHS) is characterized by frequent, repeated episodes of cyclic vomiting in individuals who chronically use cannabis.[13,71] The current literature on CHS relies almost entirely on case studies, and therefore, little is known about the prevalence or potential risk factors (eg, using high-potency cannabis or method of cannabis intake) for developing the syndrome.[72–74] The largest case series on CHS found that the average age of onset of symptoms was 25.3 years.[13] One study assessing self-reported symptoms of the syndrome in a sample of adult patients presenting to the emergency department and who also endorse currently using cannabis more than20 times per month found that 32.9% of those who used cannabis frequently met diagnostic criteria for CHS.[75] The incidence of CHS cases in emergency departments in Colorado has increased by almost 2-fold since legalization of recreational cannabis.[72,76]

The pathophysiology of CHS is unknown and still being investigated by researchers.[65,67] The Rome IV is the most recently updated tool for diagnosing CHS and was designed for use in adults.[77] An interesting clinical feature of CHS observed frequently in patients is a pattern of excessive bathing. The bathing is reported to provide relief from cyclic vomiting, and patients with CHS often spend a great deal of time seeking this relief.[13,65] Sorensen and colleagues[66] (2017) conducted a systematic review of the current literature on CHS in adults and found that 92.3% of all participants endorsed excessive bathing for relief. Weight loss also seems to be associated with CHS in some studies, although this symptom is not as commonly reported as excessive bathing.[13,67,71] The current research on CHS is mainly focused on describing the symptoms of the syndrome and possible treatments. At present, the most successful treatment is complete cessation from cannabis use, and more research is needed to determine the degree of abstinence needed to ensure continued recovery.[13,65,71]

Cannabis withdrawal syndrome occurs after cessation of cannabis use among some who use cannabis regularly. The syndrome can be diagnosed using a 15- or 22-item checklist derived from the Cannabis Withdrawal Checklist, created by Budney in 1999.[78–80] Cannabis withdrawal is marked by a wide array of physical and psychological symptoms such as anxiety, insomnia, and sweating, but most relevant to gastrointestinal function are the symptoms of nausea, stomach pain, and appetite loss. The existing literature on the topic supports the fact that women are more likely to experience these gastrointestinal-related symptoms than men.[61,63]

Finally, cannabis has been studied as a potential treatment of digestive disorders. Self-reported data support that there are individuals with inflammatory bowel disease (IBD) who have tried cannabis as a treatment and report relief from symptoms such as nausea and appetite loss.[64,68] Researchers posit that the antiinflammatory effects of cannabis are likely responsible for the symptom relief reported from cannabis use through the interaction between cannabis and the endocannabinoid system, which has receptors present across the gastrointestinal system.[81–83] Most of the research on cannabis as a treatment of IBD comes from adults; however, Hoffenberg and colleagues[62] (2019) investigated the use of cannabis oil in adolescents and young adults with IBD, also finding support for cannabis oil relieving these symptoms. This topic is still largely under investigation, and there are very few clinical trials to support cannabis as a useful treatment of gastrointestinal disorders. The existing clinical trials support that cannabis is tolerated by patients but do not conclude that it is an effective treatment of these disorders.[68–70,84,85]

ENDOCRINE FUNCTION

The existing literature focused on the effects of cannabis use on hormone function focuses almost exclusively on adults and predominantly on fertility, sexual function, hunger hormones, thyroid function, and psychobiological aspects of stress.[11,86–93] Some studies have shown that cannabis use may affect hormone levels involved in various important endocrine systems, including the hypothalamic-pituitary-adrenal (HPA) axis.[86,94] Although adolescent-focused research on this topic is scarce, increasing attention has been given to the possible effect of cannabis on pubertal timing and tempo in adolescents, informed by animal studies conducted in the 1980s and 1990s. Specifically, animal data support that prepubertal exposure to cannabis is associated with pubertal delays in women and decreases in pubertal growth spurts in men.[92,95–98]

The research focused on the effect of cannabis use on fertility and sexual function focuses heavily on men, with little conclusive evidence on women.[88–91,93,99–101] Some studies on women suggest that fertility may be decreased by cannabis use, whereas other studies have refuted any effect of cannabis on female fertility.[89,91,93,99] The current literature on the fertility and sexual function of adult men who use cannabis shows a tendency for those who used to have lower sperm counts and lower sperm concentrations compared to those who do not use cannabis.[88,90] Studies on the effect of cannabis on testosterone have mixed results, as some support heightened testosterone levels in men who use cannabis, some have seen no effects, and some support lower testosterone levels compared to men who do not use cannabis.[88,90,100,101]

Few studies have investigated the effect of cannabis use on thyroid function in humans. Existing studies have been conducted with adults, using biological measures to assess levels of the thyroid-stimulating hormone (TSH).[11,102,103] The primary role of TSH is to stimulate the thyroid gland to release triiodothyronine (T3) and thyroxine (T4). Abnormal levels of these hormones can lead to metabolic dysfunction or disease, such as hyperthyroidism and hypothyroidism.[104] Two well-designed studies pertaining to cannabis use and thyroid function were identified from the current literature and results from these studies are mixed. Bonnet (2013)[102] found no significant differences in thyroid hormone levels between adults who use cannabis compared to those who do not, whereas Malhotra and colleagues[11] (2017) found lower levels of TSH among those who use cannabis compared to those who do not. There is no evidence to support that cannabis use is associated with thyroid dysfunction at this time, but the early findings supporting the potential ability of cannabis to affect levels of key hormones such as TSH suggest more research is needed to confirm this.[11]

Cannabis has been shown to acutely increase appetite,[105,106] but research related to cannabis use and hunger hormones is limited. All empirical human studies on this topic use samples of adults and focus chiefly on insulin, ghrelin, leptin, peptide YY, and glucagon-like peptide 1.[87,107] Farokhnia and colleagues (2020) conducted a randomized, placebo-controlled trial of the effect of cannabis ingestion on various hunger-related hormones, accounting for different routes of cannabis administration. Their study found that compared to placebo, cannabis intake was associated with a decrease in the normal and expected insulin spike following sugar intake. They also found support for decreased levels of glucagon-like peptide 1. An increase in levels of ghrelin was observed, but only following oral cannabis intake.[87] Glucagon-like peptide 1 is necessary for decreasing appetite after eating, so lower levels may disrupt the body's ability to feel satiated.[108,109] Ghrelin, in contrast, is responsible for stimulating appetite, and it is logical that cannabis would appear to decrease appetite suppressing hormones and increase appetite stimulating hormones, as a substance known to increase appetite in the short-term.[87] One study among rats confirmed that cannabis use is associated with increasing ghrelin levels.[110]

Some of the most compelling findings pertaining to endocrine function and cannabis use come from studies on the effect of cannabis on stress hormones and the HPA axis. The HPA axis is responsible for the physiological response to stress, and dysfunction in the HPA axis can have negative consequences for physical and emotional health.[14,86,94,111] Few studies had samples of adolescents, and studies that had adolescent samples were either animal studies or clinical samples, such as adolescents who are at-risk for psychosis.[111,112] However, findings from a nonclinical cohort study of adolescents, the TRacking Adolescents' Individual Lives Survey (TRAILS) study, have yielded interesting results pertaining to stress reactivity and cannabis use.[14,113] Results from the TRAILS study show a tendency for decreased stress reactivity in adolescents with lifetime cannabis use compared to those who had never used cannabis, while controlling for sociodemographic contributors to stress.[14] The TRAILS study has also found that adolescents with early onset cannabis use had lower cortisol levels after waking compared to adolescents who have never used cannabis or initiated use later. In contrast, they found support for higher cortisol levels in the evening among those who endorse using cannabis at least once in their lifetime compared to those who have never used cannabis; this suggests that adolescent cannabis use, and particularly earlier initiation, may disrupt the normal cortisol fluctuations experienced throughout the day.[113] Early onset was defined as cannabis use onset between ages 9 and 12 years and later onset between ages 13 and 14 years.[113] Empirical studies addressing the use of cannabis on both psychological and physiological aspects of stress have been conducted with adults and have found a dampened stress response among those who use, even after periods of abstinence.[86,94] Data from adults have also shown that those who currently use cannabis compared to those who do not have elevated baseline levels of cortisol and adrenocorticotropic hormone compared to those who have never used cannabis, with the highest levels observed in those who currently use.[86] The observed effects of decreased stress responsiveness and general heightened stress hormone levels in these studies may show a potentially problematic effect of cannabis use on everyday functioning, but this has been refuted by some studies, suggesting that more research needs to be conducted on this topic.[114,115]

BODY MASS INDEX

Children and adolescents who are obese are more likely to have high blood pressure and cholesterol,[116] breathing problems including asthma,[117] sleep apnea,[118] and an increased risk of type 2 diabetes.[119] Thus, understanding factors that contribute to BMI in children and adolescents is an important public health issue. In particular, acute intoxication of cannabis is associated with appetite stimulation and increased caloric intake.[105,106] However, the long-term effects of cannabis use on BMI among adolescents is less clear. Results among the few studies that have been conducted on the association between these variables is mixed. Several studies have found no association between these variables,[120–122] whereas one study found that increased cannabis use during adolescence is associated with increased risk of obesity in young adulthood.[123] Another cross-sectional study found that more frequent cannabis use is associated with a higher BMI and greater likelihood of being classified as overweight or obese.[124] However, in the same sample of adolescents an increase in cannabis use was associated with a decrease in BMI.[125] The association between cannabis use and BMI has been more extensively studied among adults compared to adolescents.

Similar to the research among adolescents, studies among adults have generally reported mixed findings. For example, some research has suggested there is no association between cannabis use and BMI,[126–129] whereas other studies report a positive association between cannabis use with BMI,[124,130] abdominal fat,[131] and metabolic syndrome.[132] However, most of the studies on this topic have found a negative association between cannabis use and BMI when comparing those who use cannabis to those who do not[133–135] and when examining dose-dependent associations.[57,58,125,136] Furthermore, other factors related to BMI are also associated with cannabis use, such as lower rates and risk factors for diabetes,[135,137,138] lower likelihood of cardiometabolic diagnoses,[58,139] and smaller waist circumference.[135] Other factors related to BMI such as diet and exercise engagement may help explain the association between cannabis use and BMI.

Although cannabis use among adults is most consistently associated with a lower BMI, those who use cannabis tend to report a higher caloric intake,[140] a lower diet quality,[141] and engaging in more unhealthy weight control behaviors such as skipping meals.[142] Adults who endorsed past month cannabis use reported eating fewer vegetables and fruits compared to those who have never used or used previously. However, adults who currently use cannabis reported eating less sodium and refined grains compared to those who have never used cannabis.[141] In a prior study from 2001, those who currently use cannabis reported higher sodium intake, eating fewer fruits, and eating more salty snacks. Furthermore, those who currently use reported a higher caloric intake but still had a lower BMI.[143] In regard to exercise, adults who currently or previously used cannabis are more likely to report meeting recommended levels of exercise compared to those who have never used cannabis.[144] In addition, in one study of adults who currently use cannabis, around 80% reported using cannabis shortly before or after physical activity and these individuals reported engaging in aerobic and anerobic exercise for longer and reported greater enjoyment from exercising compared to those who do not use cannabis concurrently with exercise.[145] In line with the adult literature, one study among adolescents reported a positive association between frequency of cannabis use and greater exercise engagement.[146]

More research, particularly among adolescent samples, is needed on this topic to better understand the mechanisms through which cannabis use affects BMI. More evidence suggests that the endocannabinoid system, which contains cannabinoid type 1 (CB1) receptors and endogenous ligands, is likely involved with appetite. Δ9-THC is the primary psychoactive compound in cannabis and is a partial agonist of the CB1 receptor. Thus, a drug, Rimonabant, was developed to decrease appetite among obese individuals, acting as a selective antagonist/inverse agonist of the CB1 receptor. Rimonabant was an effective weight loss drug; however, it was denied approval by the Food and Drug Administration because of severe psychiatric side effects.[147] In summary, cannabis use is associated with a lower BMI,[57,58,125,133–136] poorer diet such as eating fewer vegetables and fruits,[140–143] and higher levels of exercise engagement.[144,145] However, more research is needed among adolescents to understand if these associations are present earlier in life and the mechanisms through which cannabis use acts on these factors.

SLEEP

Sleep is an important aspect of adolescent development, playing a crucial role in physiology, cognition, and mental health.[148,149] The endocannabinoid system is thought to be involved in the modulation of circadian rhythm and the sleep/wake cycle,[150,151] particularly through the influence of cannabinoids on CB1 receptors.[152,153] Heavy cannabis activity is linked to desensitization, and decreased CB1 efficacy[154,155] and blocking of the CB1 receptors have been found to facilitate waking in rodent models specifically.[156,157] There is limited evidence to suggest that cannabis use might influence aspects of the sleep cycle such as slow-wave sleep (SWS)[158–160] and rapid eye movement sleep.[161,162] Although cannabis is often thought to be a sleep aid[163] and there is evidence of acute cannabis use being linked to temporary sleep benefits, research implies that consistent and increased frequency of cannabis use in general is associated with sleep deficits and sleep pathology across multiple domains.[163,164]

Most existing research has been conducted in adult populations, but cross-sectional studies focused on adolescent cannabis use have found associations with various sleep factors including insomnia (defined as trouble falling asleep or staying asleep almost every day),[165] insufficient sleep on school nights,[166,167] shorter total sleep time, later bedtimes,[168] greater endorsement of past month sleep problems (eg, waking up several times per night and waking up feeling tired and worn out),[169] an evening chronotype (a preference for later sleep-wake timing),[170] and modest sleep architecture alterations at the onset of abstinence (lower percent SWS).[171] One study found differential effects with an association at baseline (mean age 15 years) between cannabis use and weekend oversleep, but an opposite relationship at follow-up (mean age 17 years) between cannabis use and lower weekend sleep duration.[172] Interestingly, we see a bidirectional association between these domains, with both early sleep problems and an evening chronotype predicting later cannabis use outcomes,[170,173,174] and earlier age of cannabis use behaviors predicting later sleep deficits and pathology such as worse sleep quality,[175] shorter sleep duration,[176,177] insomnia, and insomnia with short sleep.[178] One study found more complex associations, with higher levels of baseline weekday, and total sleep (mean age 15 years) predicted lower levels of cannabis use at a 2-year follow-up (mean age 17 years), whereas cannabis use at baseline predicted more weekend sleep, greater weekend oversleep, and higher total sleep at follow-up.[122]

With both cross-sectional and bidirectional associations, a common liability such as shared genetics could explain these associations,[177] such that the genes that contribute to cannabis use behaviors also contribute to sleep deficits (or vice versa). Evidence of an association in both directions could also be rooted in differing developmental processes. Prenatal cannabis exposure has been associated with child sleep outcomes across development. Significant differences have been found in irregular sleep, sleep-related body movements,[179] and abnormal sleep wake cycles days after birth.[180] Effects later in life have been noted, including increased nocturnal arousals, greater awake time after sleep onset, and lower sleep efficiency at age 3 years,[181] as well as increased endorsement of symptoms of sleep wake disorders, disorders of initiating and maintaining sleep, disorders of arousal, disorders of excessive somnolence, and higher sleep disorder scores at ages 9 to 10 years.[182] The fetal brain is densely populated with CB1 receptors that escalate in activity during gestation and are believed to affect brain development.[183,184] It is possible that early cannabis use or exposure could affect sleep via CB1 receptors. However, early sleep issues could lead to emotional dysregulation and cognitive deficits that could increase susceptibility to substance use and in turn lead to more sleep issues.[185]

Nevertheless, the complexities of this association are yet to be understood and research regarding cannabis use and adolescent sleep outcomes remains understudied. There are no studies to date looking specifically at the effects of CBD and THC on adolescent sleep. Research in adult populations suggest that CBD and THC have differential effects on sleep outcomes depending on the dosage. Broadly, high doses of CBD have been found to have sedating effects and low doses of CBD are associated with stimulating effects, whereas low-dose THC is thought to be sedating and high-dose/long-term THC seems to obstruct sleep.[164]

SUMMARY

Prevalence of cannabis use is high among adolescents. Daily use of cannabis was at its highest level in 2020 compared to the past 30 years, with 1.1%, 4.4%, and 6.9% of students in 8th, 10th, and 12th grade, respectively, reporting daily use of cannabis.[10] In addition, perceived harmfulness of cannabis has decreased steadily since 1991 among adolescents.[10] Furthermore, recreational and medical legalization has made cannabis more widely available across the United States among adolescents. Adolescence is a developmental period characterized by dramatic growth in physical and psychological health. As a result, it is imperative that we understand how cannabis use affects pulmonary, cardiovascular, gastrointestinal, and endocrine function and BMI and sleep during this critical developmental period.

There are some significant limitations in the current research on how cannabis use affects physical health among adolescents. Most research has primarily included adults. As a result, less is known about the physical health effects of cannabis use among adolescents. It would be important to understand how cannabis use affects the physical health of those who are already vulnerable to health issues, such as adolescents with asthma. In addition, research should focus on aspects of physical health most relevant to adolescents such as activities that involve greater cardiovascular and pulmonary strength (eg, sports and playing a wind instrument). From 1995 to 2014 in the United States, THC potency increased from 4% to 12% and the ratio of THC to CBD increased from 14:1 to 80:1 among cannabis products confiscated by law enforcement.[186] However, many people in the United States now have access to legal cannabis markets that offer high-potency cannabis concentrates that have THC levels greater than 90%. However, there is little to no research on the impact of differing cannabis potency on physical health. Perhaps results would differ in individuals using products with greater than 90% THC. In addition, there are different methods of cannabis consumption such as vaping and edibles as well as different cannabis compounds, and we do not have a good understanding of how these novel cannabis products may affect physical health among adolescents.

Overall, the extant literature suggests that cannabis use, and more frequent use, may have negative effects on physical health particularly in the domains of pulmonary function and sleep. Specifically, cannabis use is associated with coughing, wheezing, shortness of breath, and sputum production[29,32,33,37] as well as insomnia, later bedtimes, not enough sleep on school nights, and greater sleep problems.[165–169] It is less clear whether cannabis use in adolescence negatively affects diet or gastrointestinal, hormone, or cardiovascular function. Importantly, cannabis use does seem to have some rare, but serious and sometimes deadly, side effects that have been reported in adolescents and young adults. These side effects include CHS (ie, cyclic vomiting),[13,71] cardiovascular events sometimes leading to sudden death (eg, myocardial infarction, atrial fibrillation, ventricular tachycardia),[50–52] and acute lung injury leading to hospitalization and death.[45,187] More research is clearly needed to better understand how cannabis use may affect physical health during this vulnerable developmental period.

FUNDING

This work was supported by a grant from the National Institute on Drug Abuse (DA054212: J.M. Ross). The content is solely the responsibility of the authors and does not necessarily represent the official views of the National Institutes of Health. The authors have no other conflicts of interest to declare.

CONFLICT OF INTEREST

The authors do not have any conflicts of interest to declare.

CLINICS CARE POINTS

- Adolescent cannabis use is associated with coughing, wheezing, shortness of breath, and sputum production and sleep problems.

- Adolescet cannabis use is associated with several rare but serious side effects:
  - Cannabinoid hypermesis syndrome (that is cyclic vomiting)
  - Cardiovascular events (such as myocardial infarction, atrial fibilation, and ventricular tachycardia)
  - Acute lung injury (that is e-cigarette or vaping product use-associated lung injury)

REFERENCES

1. Gray KM, Squeglia LM. Research review: what have we learned about adolescent substance use? J Child Psychol Psychiatry 2018;59(6):618–27.
2. Lisdahl KM, Sher KJ, Conway KP, et al. Adolescent brain cognitive development (ABCD) study: overview of substance use assessment methods. Dev Cogn Neurosci 2018;32:80–96.
3. Patton GC, McMorris BJ, Toumbourou JW, et al. Puberty and the onset of substance use and abuse. Pediatr 2004;114(3):e300–6.

4. Carliner H, Brown QL, Sarvet AL, et al. Cannabis use, attitudes, and legal status in the US: a review. Prev Med 2017;104:13–23.

5. Lubman DI, Cheetham A, Yücel M. Cannabis and adolescent brain development. Pharmacol Ther 2015;148:1–16.

6. Meier MH, Caspi A, Ambler A, et al. Persistent cannabis users show neuropsychological decline from childhood to midlife. Proc Natl Acad Sci 2012;109(40): E2657–64.

7. Hasin DS, Shmulewitz D, Sarvet AL. Time trends in US cannabis use and cannabis use disorders overall and by sociodemographic subgroups: a narrative review and new findings. Am J Drug Alcohol Abuse 2019;45(6):623–43.

8. Sarvet AL, Wall MM, Keyes KM, et al. Recent rapid decrease in adolescents' perception that marijuana is harmful, but no concurrent increase in use. Drug Alcohol Depend 2018;186:68–74.

9. Smart R, Pacula RL. Early evidence of the impact of cannabis legalization on cannabis use, cannabis use disorder, and the use of other substances: findings from state policy evaluations. Am J Drug Alcohol Abuse 2019;45(6):644–63.

10. Johnston LD, Miech RA, O'Malley PM, et al. Monitoring the future national survey results on drug use, 1975-2020: overview, key findings on adolescent drug use. Inst Social Res 2021;1–36.

11. Malhotra S, Heptulla RA, Homel P, et al. Effect of marijuana use on thyroid function and autoimmunity. Thyroid 2017;27(2):167–73.

12. Pletcher MJ, Vittinghoff E, Kalhan R, et al. Association between marijuana exposure and pulmonary function over 20 years. JAMA 2012;307(2):173–81.

13. Simonetto DA, Oxentenko AS, Herman ML, et al. Cannabinoid hyperemesis: a case series of 98 patients. Mayo Clin Proc 2012;87(2):114–9.

14. van Leeuwen AP, Creemers HE, Greaves-Lord K, et al. Hypothalamic–pituitary-adrenal axis reactivity to social stress and adolescent cannabis use: the TRAILS study. Addiction 2011;106(8):1484–92.

15. Knapp AA, Lee DC, Borodovsky JT, et al. Emerging trends in cannabis administration among adolescent cannabis users. J Adolesc Health 2019;64(4): 487–93.

16. Kowitt SD, Osman A, Meernik C, et al. Vaping cannabis among adolescents: prevalence and associations with tobacco use from a cross-sectional study in the USA. BMJ Open 2019;9(6):e028535.

17. Trivers KF, Phillips E, Gentzke AS, et al. Prevalence of cannabis use in electronic cigarettes among US youth. JAMA Pediatr 2018;172(11):1097–9.

18. Meier MH, Docherty M, Leischow SJ, et al. Cannabis concentrate use in adolescents. Pediatr 2019;144(3):e20190338.

19. Cerdá M, Wall M, Feng T, et al. Association of state recreational marijuana laws with adolescent marijuana use. JAMA Pediatr 2017;171(2):142–9.

20. Pacula RL, Powell D, Heaton P, et al. Assessing the effects of medical marijuana laws on marijuana use: the devil is in the details. J Policy Anal Manage 2015; 34(1):7–31.

21. Wen H, Hockenberry JM, Cummings JR. The effect of medical marijuana laws on adolescent and adult use of marijuana, alcohol, and other substances. J Health Econ 2015;42:64–80.

22. Harper S, Strumpf EC, Kaufman JS. Do medical marijuana laws increase marijuana use? Replication study and extension. Ann Epidemiol 2012;22(3):207–12.

23. Lynne-Landsman SD, Livingston MD, Wagenaar AC. Effects of state medical marijuana laws on adolescent marijuana use. Am J Public Health 2013;103(8): 1500–6.

24. Wall MM, Poh E, Cerdá M, et al. Adolescent marijuana use from 2002 to 2008: higher in states with medical marijuana laws, cause still unclear. Ann Epidemiol 2011;21(9):714–6.

25. Aldington S, Harwood M, Cox B, et al. Cannabis use and risk of lung cancer: a case–control study. Eur Respir J 2008;31(2):280–6.

26. Aldington S, Williams M, Nowitz M, et al. Effects of cannabis on pulmonary structure, function and symptoms. Thorax 2007;62(12):1058–63.

27. Hancox RJ, Poulton R, Ely M, et al. Effects of cannabis on lung function: a population-based cohort study. Eur Respir J 2010;35(1):42–7.

28. Taylor DR, Fergusson DM, Milne BJ, et al. A longitudinal study of the effects of tobacco and cannabis exposure on lung function in young adults. Addiction 2002;97(8):1055–61.

29. Taylor DR, Poulton R, Moffitt TE, et al. The respiratory effects of cannabis dependence in young adults. Addiction 2000;95(11):1669–77.

30. Winhusen T, Theobald J, Kaelber DC, et al. Regular cannabis use, with and without tobacco co-use, is associated with respiratory disease. Drug Alcohol Depend 2019;204:107557.

31. Bramness JG, von Soest T. A longitudinal study of cannabis use increasing the use of asthma medication in young Norwegian adults. BMC Pulm Med 2019; 19(1):1–7.

32. Macleod J, Robertson R, Copeland L, et al. Cannabis, tobacco smoking, and lung function: a cross-sectional observational study in a general practice population. Br J Gen Pract 2015;65(631):e89–95.

33. Moore BA, Augustson EM, Moser RP, et al. Respiratory effects of marijuana and tobacco use in a US sample. J Gen Intern Med 2005;20(1):33–7.

34. Krishnasamy VP, Hallowell BD, Ko JY, et al. Update: characteristics of a nationwide outbreak of e-cigarette, or vaping, product use–associated lung injury— United States, August 2019–January 2020. MMWR Surveill Summ 2020; 69(3):90.

35. Lozier MJ, Wallace B, Anderson K, et al. Update: demographic, product, and substance-use characteristics of hospitalized patients in a Nationwide outbreak of E-cigarette, or Vaping, product use–associated lung injuries—United States, December 2019. MMWR Surveill Summ 2019;68(49):1142.

36. Thakrar PD, Boyd KP, Swanson CP, et al. E-cigarette, or vaping, product use-associated lung injury in adolescents: a review of imaging features. Pediatr Radiol 2020;50(3):338–44.

37. Tetrault JM, Crothers K, Moore BA, et al. Effects of marijuana smoking on pulmonary function and respiratory complications: a systematic review. Arch Intern Med 2007;167(3):221–8.

38. Eschenbacher WL. Defining airflow obstruction. Chronic Obstr Pulm Dis 2016; 3(2):515.

39. Heckman EJ, O'Connor GT. Pulmonary function tests for diagnosing lung disease. JAMA 2015;313(22):2278–9.

40. Yayan J, Rasche K. Damaging effects of cannabis use on the lungs. Adv Clin Res 2016;952:31–4.

41. Callaghan RC, Allebeck P, Sidorchuk A. Marijuana use and risk of lung cancer: a 40-year cohort study. Cancer Causes Control 2013;24(10):1811–20.

42. Tan WC, Lo C, Jong A, et al. Marijuana and chronic obstructive lung disease: a population-based study. CMAJ 2009;180(8):814–20.

43. Gracie K, Hancox RJ. Cannabis use disorder and the lungs. Addiction 2021; 116(1):182–90.

44. Tashkin DP, Simmons MS, Tseng C-H. Impact of changes in regular use of marijuana and/or tobacco on chronic bronchitis. COPD 2012;9(4):367–74.
45. Cherian SV, Kumar A, Estrada-Y-Martin RM. E-cigarette or vaping product-associated lung injury: a review. Am J Med 2020;133(6):657–63.
46. Winnicka L, Shenoy MA. EVALI and the pulmonary toxicity of electronic cigarettes: a review. J Gen Intern Med 2020;35(7):2130–5.
47. Werner AK, Koumans EH, Chatham-Stephens K, et al. Hospitalizations and deaths associated with EVALI. N Engl J Med 2020;382(17):1589–98.
48. Menkes DB, Howard RC, Spears GF, et al. Salivary THC following cannabis smoking correlates with subjective intoxication and heart rate. Psychopharmacol 1991;103(2):277–9.
49. Volavka J, Crown P, Dornbush R, et al. EEG, heart rate and mood change ("high") after cannabis. Psychopharmacologia 1973;32(1):11–25.
50. Bachs L, Mørland H. Acute cardiovascular fatalities following cannabis use. Forensic Sci Int 2001;124(2–3):200–3.
51. Mittleman MA, Lewis RA, Maclure M, et al. Triggering myocardial infarction by marijuana. Circ 2001;103(23):2805–9.
52. Rezkalla S, Kloner RA. Cardiovascular effects of marijuana. Trends Cardiovasc Med 2019;29(7):403–7.
53. Schmid K, Schönlebe J, Drexler H, et al. The effects of cannabis on heart rate variability and well-being in young men. Pharmacopsychiatry 2010;43(04):147–50.
54. Ross JM, Ellingson JM, Frieser MJ. The effects of cannabis use on physical health: a co-twin control study. Drug and Alcohol Depend 2021;230:109200.
55. Graham J, Li D. Cardiovascular and respiratory effects of cannabis in cat and rat. Br J Pharmacol 1973;49(1):1–10.
56. Alshaarawy O, Elbaz HA. Cannabis use and blood pressure levels: United States national health and nutrition examination survey, 2005–2012. J Hypertens 2016;34(8):1507.
57. Meier MH, Caspi A, Cerdá M, et al. Associations between cannabis use and physical health problems in early midlife: a longitudinal comparison of persistent cannabis vs tobacco users. JAMA Psychiatry 2016;73(7):731–40.
58. Meier MH, Pardini D, Beardslee J, et al. Associations between cannabis use and cardiometabolic risk factors: a longitudinal study of men. Psychosom Med 2019;81(3):281–8.
59. Bonnet U. Abrupt quitting of long-term heavy recreational cannabis use is not followed by significant changes in blood pressure and heart rate. Pharmacopsychiatry 2016;49(01):23–5.
60. Vandrey R, Umbricht A, Strain EC. Increased blood pressure following abrupt cessation of daily cannabis use. J Addict Med 2011;5(1):16.
61. Herrmann ES, Weerts EM, Vandrey R. Sex differences in cannabis withdrawal symptoms among treatment-seeking cannabis users. Exp Clin Psychopharmacol 2015;23(6):415.
62. Hoffenberg EJ, McWilliams S, Mikulich-Gilbertson S, et al. Cannabis oil use by adolescents and young adults with inflammatory bowel disease. J Pediatr Gastroenterol Nutr 2019;68(3):348–52.
63. Preuss U, Watzke A, Zimmermann J, et al. Cannabis withdrawal severity and short-term course among cannabis-dependent adolescent and young adult inpatients. Drug Alcohol Depend 2010;106(2–3):133–41.
64. Goyal H, Singla U, Gupta U, et al. Role of cannabis in digestive disorders. Eur J Gastroenterol Hepatol 2017;29(2):135–43.

65. Sawni A, Vaniawala VP, Good M, et al. Recurrent cyclic vomiting in adolescents: can it be cannabinoid hyperemesis syndrome? Clin Pediatr 2016;55(6):560–3.
66. Sorensen CJ, DeSanto K, Borgelt L, et al. Cannabinoid hyperemesis syndrome: diagnosis, pathophysiology, and treatment—a systematic review. J Med Toxicol 2017;13(1):71–87.
67. Zhu JW, Gonsalves CL, Issenman RM, et al. Diagnosis and acute management of adolescent cannabinoid hyperemesis syndrome: a systematic review. J Adolesc Health 2021;68(2):246–54.
68. Gotfried J, Naftali T, Schey R. Role of cannabis and its derivatives in gastrointestinal and hepatic disease. Gastroenterol 2020;159(1):62–80.
69. Irving PM, Iqbal T, Nwokolo C, et al. A randomized, double-blind, placebo-controlled, parallel-group, pilot study of cannabidiol-rich botanical extract in the symptomatic treatment of ulcerative colitis. Inflamm Bowel Dis 2018;24(4): 714–24.
70. Kafil TS, Nguyen TM, MacDonald JK, et al. Cannabis for the treatment of crohn's disease and ulcerative colitis: evidence from Cochrane Reviews. Inflamm Bowel Dis 2020;26(4):502–9.
71. Allen J, De Moore G, Heddle R, et al. Cannabinoid hyperemesis: cyclical hyperemesis in association with chronic cannabis abuse. Gut 2004;53(11):1566–70.
72. DeVuono MV, Parker LA. Cannabinoid hyperemesis syndrome: a review of potential mechanisms. Cannabis Cannabinoid Res 2020;5(2):132–44.
73. Fleming JE, Lockwood S. Cannabinoid hyperemesis syndrome. Fed Pract 2017; 34(10):33.
74. Khattar N, Routsolias JC. Emergency department treatment of cannabinoid hyperemesis syndrome: a review. Am J Ther 2018;25(3):e357–61.
75. Habboushe J, Rubin A, Liu H, et al. The prevalence of cannabinoid hyperemesis syndrome among regular marijuana smokers in an urban public hospital. Basic Clin Pharmacol Toxicol 2018;122(6):660–2.
76. Kim HS, Anderson JD, Saghafi O, et al. Cyclic vomiting presentations following marijuana liberalization in Colorado. Acad Emerg Med 2015;22(6):694–9.
77. Stanghellini V, Chan FK, Hasler WL, et al. Gastroduodenal disorders. Gastroenterol 2016;150(6):1380–92.
78. American Psychological Association. Diagnostic and statistical manual of mental disorders (DSM-5®). Washington, DC: American Psychiatric Pub; 2013.
79. Bonnet U, Preuss UW. The cannabis withdrawal syndrome: current insights. Subst Abuse Rehabil 2017;8:9.
80. Budney AJ, Novy PL, Hughes JR. Marijuana withdrawal among adults seeking treatment for marijuana dependence. Addiction 1999;94(9):1311–22.
81. DiPatrizio NV. Endocannabinoids in the gut. Cannabis Cannabinoid Res 2016; 1(1):67–77.
82. Izzo AA, Sharkey KA. Cannabinoids and the gut: new developments and emerging concepts. Pharmacol Ther 2010;126(1):21–38.
83. Picardo S, Kaplan GG, Sharkey KA, et al. Insights into the role of cannabis in the management of inflammatory bowel disease. Therap Adv Gastroenterol 2019; 12. 1756284819870977.
84. Naftali T, Mechulam R, Marii A, et al. Low-dose cannabidiol is safe but not effective in the treatment for Crohn's disease, a randomized controlled trial. Dig Dis Sci 2017;62(6):1615–20.
85. Naftali T, Schleider LB-L, Dotan I, et al. Cannabis induces a clinical response in patients with Crohn's disease: a prospective placebo-controlled study. Clin Gastroenterol Hepatol 2013;11(10):1276–80. e1.

86. Cuttler C, Spradlin A, Nusbaum AT, et al. Blunted stress reactivity in chronic cannabis users. Psychopharmacol 2017;234(15):2299–309.

87. Farokhnia M, McDiarmid GR, Newmeyer MN, et al. Effects of oral, smoked, and vaporized cannabis on endocrine pathways related to appetite and metabolism: a randomized, double-blind, placebo-controlled, human laboratory study. Transl Psychiatry 2020;10(1):1–11.

88. Gundersen TD, Jørgensen N, Andersson A-M, et al. Association between use of marijuana and male reproductive hormones and semen quality: a study among 1,215 healthy young men. Am J Epidemiol 2015;182(6):473–81.

89. Kasman AM, Thoma ME, McLain AC, et al. Association between use of marijuana and time to pregnancy in men and women: findings from the National Survey of Family Growth. Fertil Steril 2018;109(5):866–71.

90. Kolodny RC, Masters WH, Kolodner RM, et al. Depression of plasma testosterone levels after chronic intensive marihuana use. N Engl J Med 1974; 290(16):872–4.

91. Mumford S, Flannagan K, Radoc J, et al. Cannabis use while trying to conceive: a prospective cohort study evaluating associations with fecundability, live birth and pregnancy loss. Hum Reprod 2021;36(5):1405–15.

92. Sims ED, Anvari S, Lee Y, et al. The effect of cannabis exposure on pubertal outcomes: a systematic review. Adolesc Health Med Ther 2018;9:137.

93. Wise LA, Wesselink AK, Hatch EE, et al. Marijuana use and fecundability in a North American preconception cohort study. J Epidemiol Community Health 2018;72(3):208–15.

94. Somaini L, Manfredini M, Amore M, et al. Psychobiological responses to unpleasant emotions in cannabis users. Eur Arch Psychiatry Clin Neurosci 2012; 262(1):47–57.

95. Field E, Tyrey L. Delayed sexual maturation in the female rat during chronic exposure to delta-9-tetrahydrocannabinol. Life Sci 1984;35(17):1725–30.

96. Field E, Tyrey L. Delayed sexual maturation during prepubertal cannabinoid treatment: importance of the timing of treatment. J Pharmacol Exp Ther 1990; 254(1):171–5.

97. Gupta D, Elbracht C. Effect of tetrahydrocannabinols on pubertal body weight spurt and sex hormones in developing male rats. Res Exp Med 1983;182(2): 95–104.

98. Wenger T, Croix D, Tramu G. The effect of chronic prepubertal administration of marihuana (delta-9-tetrahydrocannabinol) on the onset of puberty and the postpubertal reproductive functions in female rats. Biol Reprod 1988;39(3):540–5.

99. Klonoff-Cohen HS, Natarajan L, Chen RV. A prospective study of the effects of female and male marijuana use on in vitro fertilization (IVF) and gamete intrafallopian transfer (GIFT) outcomes. Am J Obstet Gynecol 2006;194(2):369–76.

100. Mendelson JH, Kuehnle J, Ellingboe J, et al. Plasma testosterone levels before, during and after chronic marihuana smoking. N Engl J Med 1974;291(20): 1051–5.

101. Thistle JE, Graubard BI, Braunlin M, et al. Marijuana use and serum testosterone concentrations among US males. Andrology 2017;5(4):732–8.

102. Bonnet U. Chronic cannabis abuse, delta-9-tetrahydrocannabinol and thyroid function. Pharmacopsychiatry 2013;46(01):35–6.

103. Meah F, Lundholm M, Emanuele N, et al. The effects of cannabis and cannabinoids on the endocrine system. Rev Endocr Metab Disord 2021;1–20.

104. Pirahanchi Y, Tariq MA, Jialal I. In: Physiology, Thyroid. Florida: Statpearls Publishing; 2021.

105. Foltin RW, Fischman MW, Byrne MF. Effects of smoked marijuana on food intake and body weight of humans living in a residential laboratory. Appetite 1988; 11(1):1–14.

106. Green B, Kavanagh D, Young R. Being stoned: a review of self-reported cannabis effects. Drug Alcohol Rev 2003;22(4):453–60.

107. Riggs PK, Vaida F, Rossi SS, et al. A pilot study of the effects of cannabis on appetite hormones in HIV-infected adult men. Brain Res 2012;1431:46–52.

108. Müller TD, Finan B, Bloom S, et al. Glucagon-like peptide 1 (GLP-1). Mol Metab 2019;30:72–130.

109. van Bloemendaal L, IJzerman RG, Jennifer S, et al. GLP-1 receptor activation modulates appetite-and reward-related brain areas in humans. Diabetes 2014;63(12):4186–96.

110. Mazidi M, Taraghdari SB, Rezaee P, et al. The effect of hydroalcoholic extract of Cannabis Sativa on appetite hormone in rat. J Complement Integr Med 2014; 11(4):253–7.

111. Carol EE, Spencer RL, Mittal VA. The relationship between cannabis use and cortisol levels in youth at ultra high-risk for psychosis. Psychoneuroendocrinology 2017;83:58–64.

112. Schramm-Sapyta NL, Cha YM, Chaudhry S, et al. Differential anxiogenic, aversive, and locomotor effects of THC in adolescent and adult rats. Psychopharmacol 2007;191(4):867–77.

113. Huizink AC, Ferdinand RF, Ormel J, et al. Hypothalamic–pituitary–adrenal axis activity and early onset of cannabis use. Addiction 2006;101(11):1581–8.

114. Cloak CC, Alicata D, Ernst TM, et al. Psychiatric symptoms, salivary cortisol and cytokine levels in young marijuana users. J Neuroimmune Pharmacol 2015; 10(2):380–90.

115. Lisano JK, Kisiolek JN, Smoak P, et al. Chronic cannabis use and circulating biomarkers of neural health, stress, and inflammation in physically active individuals. Appl Physiol Nutr Metab 2020;45(3):258–63.

116. Cote AT, Harris KC, Panagiotopoulos C, et al. Childhood obesity and cardiovascular dysfunction. J Am Coll Cardiol 2013;62(15):1309–19.

117. Mohanan S, Tapp H, McWilliams A, et al. Obesity and asthma: pathophysiology and implications for diagnosis and management in primary care. Exp Biol Med 2014;239(11):1531–40.

118. Narang I, Mathew JL. Childhood obesity and obstructive sleep apnea. J Clin Nutr Metab 2012;2012:1–8.

119. Lloyd L, Langley-Evans S, McMullen S. Childhood obesity and risk of the adult metabolic syndrome: a systematic review. Int J Obes 2012;36(1):1–11.

120. Lanza HI, Grella CE, Chung PJ. Does adolescent weight status predict problematic substance use patterns? Am J Health Behav 2014;38(5):708–16.

121. Pasch KE, Nelson MC, Lytle LA, et al. Adoption of risk-related factors through early adolescence: associations with weight status and implications for causal mechanisms. J Adolesc Health 2008;43(4):387–93.

122. Pasch KE, Velazquez CE, Cance JD, et al. Youth substance use and body composition: does risk in one area predict risk in the other? J Youth Adolesc 2012;41(1):14–26.

123. Huang DY, Lanza HI, Anglin MD. Association between adolescent substance use and obesity in young adulthood: a group-based dual trajectory analysis. Addict Behav 2013;38(11):2653–60.

124. Ross J, Graziano P, Pacheco-Colón I, et al. Decision-making does not moderate the association between cannabis use and body mass index among adolescent cannabis users. J Int Neuropsychol Soc 2016;22(9):944–9.

125. Ross JM, Pacheco-Colón I, Hawes SW, et al. Bidirectional longitudinal associations between cannabis use and body mass index among adolescents. Cannabis Cannabinoid Res 2020;5(1):81–8.

126. Barry D, Petry NM. Associations between body mass index and substance use disorders differ by gender: results from the National Epidemiologic Survey on Alcohol and Related Conditions. Addict Behav 2009;34(1):51–60.

127. Jin LZ, Rangan A, Mehlsen J, et al. Association between use of cannabis in adolescence and weight change into midlife. PLoS One 2017;12(1):e0168897.

128. Levendal R, Schumann D, Donath M, et al. Cannabis exposure associated with weight reduction and β-cell protection in an obese rat model. Phytomedicine 2012;19(7):575–82.

129. Rooke SE, Norberg MM, Copeland J, et al. Health outcomes associated with long-term regular cannabis and tobacco smoking. Addict Behav 2013;38(6): 2207–13.

130. Liemburg EJ, Bruins J, van Beveren N, et al. Cannabis and a lower BMI in psychosis: what is the role of AKT1? Schizophr Res 2016;176(2–3):95–9.

131. Muniyappa R, Sable S, Ouwerkerk R, et al. Metabolic effects of chronic cannabis smoking. Diabetes Care 2013;36(8):2415–22.

132. Yankey BN, Strasser S, Okosun IS. A cross-sectional analysis of the association between marijuana and cigarette smoking with metabolic syndrome among adults in the United States. Diabetes Metab Syndr 2016;10(2):S89–95.

133. Danielsson A, Lundin A, Yaregal A, et al. Cannabis use as risk or protection for type 2 diabetes: a longitudinal study of 18 000 Swedish men and women. J Diabetes Res 2016;2016.

134. Gerberich SG, Sidney S, Braun BL, et al. Marijuana use and injury events resulting in hospitalization. Ann Epidemiol 2003;13(4):230–7.

135. Penner EA, Buettner H, Mittleman MA. The impact of marijuana use on glucose, insulin, and insulin resistance among US adults. Am J Med 2013;126(7):583–9.

136. Hayatbakhsh MR, O'Callaghan MJ, Mamun AA, et al. Cannabis use and obesity and young adults. Am J Drug Alcohol Abuse 2010;36(6):350–6.

137. Alshaarawy O, Anthony JC. Cannabis smoking and diabetes mellitus: results from meta-analysis with eight independent replication samples. Epidemiol 2015;26(4):597.

138. Ngueta G, Bélanger RE, Laouan-Sidi EA, et al. Cannabis use in relation to obesity and insulin resistance in the inuit population. Obesity 2015;23(2):290–5.

139. Waterreus A, Di Prinzio P, Watts GF, et al. Metabolic syndrome in people with a psychotic illness: is cannabis protective? Psychol Med 2016;46(8):1651–62.

140. Rodondi N, Pletcher MJ, Liu K, et al. Marijuana use, diet, body mass index, and cardiovascular risk factors (from the CARDIA study). Am J Cardiol 2006;98(4): 478–84.

141. Gelfand AR, Tangney CC. Dietary quality differs among cannabis use groups: data from the National Health and Nutrition Examination Survey 2005–16. Public Health Nutr 2021;24(11):3419–27.

142. Korn L, Haynie DL, Luk JW, et al. Prospective associations between cannabis use and negative and positive health and social measures among emerging adults. Int J Drug Policy 2018;58:55–63.

143. Smit E, Crespo CJ. Dietary intake and nutritional status of US adult marijuana users: results from the Third National Health and Nutrition Examination Survey. Public Health Nutr 2001;4(3):781–6.

144. Rajavashisth TB, Shaheen M, Norris KC, et al. Decreased prevalence of diabetes in marijuana users: cross-sectional data from the National Health and Nutrition Examination Survey (NHANES) III. BMJ Open 2012;2(1):e000494.

145. YorkWilliams SL, Gust CJ, Mueller R, et al. The new runner's high? Examining relationships between cannabis use and exercise behavior in states with legalized cannabis. Front Public Health 2019;7:99.

146. Pacheco-Colón I, Salamanca MJ, Coxe S, et al. Exercise, Decision-making, and cannabis-related outcomes among adolescents. Subst Use Misuse 2021;56(7): 1035–44.

147. Christensen R, Kristensen PK, Bartels EM, et al. Efficacy and safety of the weight-loss drug rimonabant: a meta-analysis of randomised trials. Lancet 2007;370(9600):1706–13.

148. Brand S, Kirov R. Sleep and its importance in adolescence and in common adolescent somatic and psychiatric conditions. Int J Gen Med 2011;4.425.

149. Tarokh L, Saletin JM, Carskadon MA. Sleep in adolescence: physiology, cognition and mental health. Neurosci Biobehav Rev 2016;70:182.

150. Murillo-Rodríguez E, Poot-Ake A, Arias-Carrión O, et al. The emerging role of the endocannabinoid system in the sleep-wake cycle modulation. Cent Nerv Syst Agents Med Chem 2011;11(3):189–96.

151. Prospéro-García O, Amancio-Belmont O, Meléndez ALB, et al. Endocannabinoids and sleep. Neurosci Biobehav Rev 2016;71:671–9.

152. Murillo-Rodríguez E. The role of the CB1 receptor in the regulation of sleep. Prog Neuropsychopharmacol Biol Psychiatry 2008;32(6):1420–7.

153. Murillo-Rodríguez E, Machado S, Rocha NB, et al. Revealing the role of the endocannabinoid system modulators, SR141716A, URB597 and VDM-11, in sleep homeostasis. Neurosci 2016;339:433–49.

154. González S, Cebeira M, Fernández-Ruiz J. Cannabinoid tolerance and dependence: a review of studies in laboratory animals. Pharmacol Biochem Behav 2005;81(2):300–18.

155. Hirvonen J, Goodwin R, Li C-T, et al. Reversible and regionally selective down-regulation of brain cannabinoid CB 1 receptors in chronic daily cannabis smokers. Mol Psychiatry 2012;17(6):642–9.

156. Bogáthy E, Papp N, Tóthfalusi L, et al. Additive effect of 5-HT2C and CB1 receptor blockade on the regulation of sleep–wake cycle. BMC Neurosci 2019; 20(1):1–8.

157. Santucci V, Storme J-j, Soubrié P, et al. Arousal-enhancing properties of the CB1 cannabinoid receptor antagonist SR 141716A in rats as assessed by electroencephalographic spectral and sleep-waking cycle analysis. Life Sci 1996;58(6): PL103–10.

158. Barratt ES, Beaver W, White R. The effects of marijuana on human sleep patterns. Biol Psychiatry 1974;8(1):47–54.

159. Bolla KI, Lesage SR, Gamaldo CE, et al. Sleep disturbance in heavy marijuana users. Sleep 2008;31(6):901–8.

160. Nicholson AN, Turner C, Stone BM, et al. Effect of Δ-9-tetrahydrocannabinol and cannabidiol on nocturnal sleep and early-morning behavior in young adults. J Clin Psychopharmacol 2004;24(3):305–13.

161. Feinberg I, Jones R, Walker JM, et al. Effects of high dosage delta-9-tetrahydrocannabinol on sleep patterns in man. Clin Pharmacol Ther 1975; 17(4):458–66.

162. Pivik R, Zarcone V, Dement W, et al. Delta-9-tetrahydrocannabinol and synhexl: effects on human sleep patterns. Clin Pharmacol Ther 1972;13(3):426–35.

163. Altman BR, Mian M, Slavin M, et al. Cannabis expectancies for sleep. J Psychoactive Drugs 2019;51(5):405–12.

164. Edwards D, Filbey FM. Are sweet dreams made of these? Understanding the relationship between sleep and cannabis use. Cannabis Cannabinoid Res 2021;6(6):462–73.

165. Roane BM, Taylor DJ. Adolescent insomnia as a risk factor for early adult depression and substance abuse. Sleep 2008;31(10):1351–6.

166. Kwon M, Seo YS, Park E, et al. Association between substance use and insufficient sleep in US high school students. J Sch Nurs 2020;37(6). 1059840519901161.

167. McKnight-Eily LR, Eaton DK, Lowry R, et al. Relationships between hours of sleep and health-risk behaviors in US adolescent students. Prev Med 2011; 53(4–5):271–3.

168. Troxel WM, Ewing B, D'Amico EJ. Examining racial/ethnic disparities in the association between adolescent sleep and alcohol or marijuana use. Sleep Health 2015;1(2):104–8.

169. Zhabenko O, Austic E, Conroy DA, et al. Substance use as a risk factor for sleep problems among adolescents presenting to the emergency department. J Addict Med 2016;10(5):331.

170. Hasler BP, Franzen PL, de Zambotti M, et al. Eveningness and later sleep timing are associated with greater risk for alcohol and marijuana use in adolescence: initial findings from the National Consortium on Alcohol and Neurodevelopment in Adolescence Study. Alcohol Clin Exp Res 2017;41(6):1154–65.

171. Cohen-Zion M, Drummond SP, Padula CB, et al. Sleep architecture in adolescent marijuana and alcohol users during acute and extended abstinence. Addict Beh 2009;34(11):976–9.

172. Pasch KE, Latimer LA, Cance JD, et al. Longitudinal bi-directional relationships between sleep and youth substance use. J Youth Adolesc 2012;41(9):1184–96.

173. Mike TB, Shaw DS, Forbes EE, et al. The hazards of bad sleep—sleep duration and quality as predictors of adolescent alcohol and cannabis use. Drug Alcohol Depend 2016;168:335–9.

174. Wong MM, Brower KJ, Zucker RA. Childhood sleep problems, early onset of substance use and behavioral problems in adolescence. Sleep Med 2009; 10(7):787–96.

175. McPherson KL, Tomasi DG, Wang G-J, et al. Cannabis affects cerebellar volume and sleep differently in men and women. Front Psychiatry 2021;12:12.

176. Winiger EA, Huggett SB, Hatoum AS, et al. Onset of regular cannabis use and adult sleep duration: genetic variation and the implications of a predictive relationship. Drug Alcohol Depend 2019;204:107517.

177. Winiger EA, Ellingson JM, Morrison CL, et al. Sleep deficits and cannabis use behaviors: an analysis of shared genetics using linkage disequilibrium score regression and polygenic risk prediction. Sleep 2021;44(3):zsaa188.

178. Winiger EA, Huggett SB, Hatoum AS, et al. Onset of regular cannabis use and young adult insomnia: an analysis of shared genetic liability. Sleep 2020;43(5): zsz293.

179. Scher MS, Richardson GA, Coble PA, et al. The effects of prenatal alcohol and marijuana exposure: disturbances in neonatal sleep cycling and arousal. Pediatr Res 1988;24(1):101–5.
180. Pollack R, Rana D, Purvis J, et al. Effect of prenatal marijuana exposure on sleep wake cycles and amplitude-integrated electroencephalogram (aEEG). J Perinatol 2021;41(6):1–9.
181. Aarons GA, Brown SA, Coe MT, et al. Adolescent alcohol and drug abuse and health. J Adolesc Health 1999;24(6):412–21.
182. Winiger EA, Hewitt JK. Prenatal cannabis exposure and sleep outcomes in children 9–10 years of age in the adolescent brain cognitive development SM study. Sleep Health 2020;6(6):787–9.
183. Harkany T, Guzman M, Galve-Roperh I, et al. The emerging functions of endocannabinoid signaling during CNS development. Trends Pharmacol Sci 2007; 28(2):83–92.
184. Tortoriello G, Morris CV, Alpar A, et al. Miswiring the brain: Δ9-tetrahydrocannabinol disrupts cortical development by inducing an SCG 10/stathmin-2 degradation pathway. EMBO J 2014;33(7):668–85.
185. Edwards S, Reeves GM, Fishbein D. Integrative model of the relationship between sleep problems and risk for youth substance use. Curr Addict Rep 2015;2(2):130–40.
186. ElSohly MA, Mehmedic Z, Foster S, et al. Changes in cannabis potency over the last 2 decades (1995–2014): analysis of current data in the United States. Biol Psychiatry 2016;79(7):613–9.
187. Hall W, Gartner C, Bonevski B. Lessons from the public health responses to the US outbreak of vaping-related lung injury. Addiction 2021;116(5):985–93.

A Pragmatic Clinical Approach to Substance Abuse Prevention

Paula Riggs, MD

KEYWORDS

- Adolescents • Cannabis • Prevention • Substance use disorders • Resilience
- Risk factors

KEY POINTS

This article draws on 3 lines of research to

- Identify a small set of core skills deficits in young children that predict the development of substance use, serious behavior, and mental health problems by adolescence.
- identify common components of evidence-based prevention interventions that can be practically used as prevention tools without the need for additional specialized training.
- identify existing community-based prevention resources and services that can be used to enhance protective factors that foster resilience in "at-risk" youth and families.

INTRODUCTION

Substance abuse and other problem behaviors that arise during adolescence have their roots in developmental risk factors and mental health problems that occur earlier. Substance use during adolescence is associated with poor academic performance, increased school drop-out rates, and increased risk of progressing to more severe and chronic addiction.[1,2] In the expanding legalized cannabis environment, the use of high-potency cannabis products among adolescents is particularly concerning. There is growing evidence that regular cannabis use during adolescence is associated with persistent neurocognitive deficits and a greater risk of psychosis, anxiety disorders, depression, and suicidality.[2] Clinicians, families, and communities need guidance and practical approaches to support prevention and early interventions to mitigate risk factors for adolescent substance abuse and associated mental health problems.

This article originally appeared in *Child and Adolescent Psychiatric Clinics*, Volume 32 Issue 1, January 2023.
Division of Addiction Science, Prevention & Treatment, Department of Psychiatry, University of Colorado School of Medicine, Anschutz Health Sciences Building (AHSB), 1890 N Revere Court, Aurora, CO 80045, USA
E-mail address: paula.riggs@cuanschutz.edu

Psychiatr Clin N Am 46 (2023) 741–748
https://doi.org/10.1016/j.psc.2023.03.002
0193-953X/23/© 2023 Elsevier Inc. All rights reserved.

Over the past 3 decades, research has led to the development of hundreds of prevention interventions that have been shown to improve academic performance, facilitate healthy choices, and reduce the risk of developing substance abuse and mental health problems during adolescence.[1–5] Unfortunately, numerous challenges to the widespread adoption and implementation of these interventions remain. In addition, most are school-based prevention programs with limited utility in pediatric primary care or outpatient child/adolescent behavioral health treatment settings, which are ideal settings but are currently underutilized for prevention and early intervention. The main goals of this article are to (1) identify a small group of antecedent risk factors and skills deficits in young children that predict the development of substance abuse and other adverse outcomes by adolescence; (2) identify prevention tools and skills derived from evidence-based prevention interventions that can be used by a broad range of clinicians without the need for additional specialized training; and (3) identify a common core of protective factors that longitudinal studies have found to be associated with resilience and their application to prevention and early intervention.

What Can We Learn from Longitudinal Studies of Resilience?

The dozen or so longitudinal epidemiologic studies that have followed individuals from infancy to adulthood have consistently shown that even among children exposed to multiple stressors and adversities, only a minority develop serious emotional disturbances or persistent behavior problems.[6–9] Although these studies have examined different populations, a common core of protective factors can be identified across studies that seem to facilitate positive adaptations that promote resilience even in the context of adversity.[6–9] One of the longest and most informative of these studies is the Kauai Longitudinal Study, which examines the impact of a variety of biological and psychosocial risk factors and stressful life events in a multiracial cohort of 698 children born on this Hawaiian island in 1955.[6,7] This birth cohort was repeatedly assessed at ages 1, 2, 10, 18, 32, and 40 years—ages that mark the development of trust, autonomy, industry, identity, intimacy, and generativity. Approximately one-third of the total cohort (n = 210) had multiple risk factors that predict the development of substance use and serious behavior problems by adolescence. About two-thirds of this "high-risk" cohort developed learning and behavioral problems by age 10 years and had mental health problems and some involvement with the juvenile justice system by age 18 years. However, approximately one-third of the "high-risk" cohort did not develop learning or behavioral problems during childhood or adolescence. As a group, they were successful in school and adept at managing home and social life and most developed into confident, competent, and caring adults. Remarkably, by age 40 years, none were unemployed or involved with social services or had legal problems. Their divorce rates, mortality, and chronic health problems were significantly lower than other at-risk peers and were comparable to the "low-risk" cohort. Their accomplishments were also equal to or even exceeded those of the "low-risk" cohort who were raised in economically secure and stable home environments.[6,7]

As infants, the resilient subgroup was described as affectionate, cuddly, and with an easy temperament that elicited positive responses from adult caretakers. Resilient toddlers were characterized as agreeable, cheerful, friendly, responsive, and sociable. Compared with "at-risk" youth with developmental delays, resilient preschoolers demonstrated greater behavioral control and more advanced language, reading, and self-help skills that contributed to greater social competence during the transition to elementary school. By age 10 years, those from the resilient subgroup were better readers, had higher-level practical problem-solving skills, and willing to assist others who needed help. They were often involved in activities that fostered the development of special skills and talents that instilled a sense of pride. By late adolescence, resilient teens had a strong sense of self and a belief in their ability to overcome problems. As a group, they also had higher expectations for the future compared with "at-risk" peers.[6,7]

Family factors associated with resilience included a close bond with at least one competent and emotionally stable person who was sensitive to their needs. Resilient youths were skilled at recruiting "surrogate parents" or other caregivers, including grandparents, older siblings, aunts, and uncles, who provided much of their nurturing during childhood and adolescence. Resilient youths also tended to rely on elders or older peers (eg, teachers, parents of friends, youth leaders, or ministers) in their community, often seeking their counsel in times of crisis.[6,7] Families of resilient children tended to hold religious beliefs that provided stability and meaning in their lives. Resilient boys lived in households with structure and rules and often, a male role model who encouraged emotional expressiveness. Resilient girls were supported by a reliable female caregiver and often raised in families with a combined emphasis on cooperation and independence.[6,7] Resilient young adults often took advantage of "second-chance" educational or vocational training opportunities (eg, community college) that became important turning points supporting a more positive adult developmental trajectory. Most of the resilient subgroup were married to an empathic and supportive partner by young adulthood into mid-life.[6,7]

This developmental narrative from the Kauai Longitudinal Study reveals a relatively small set of protective skills and individual characteristics that promoted resilience in a subgroup of "at-risk" youth. Compared with other "at-risk" peers, the resilient subgroup had greater behavioral control, more advanced language, reading skills, and self-help skills that contributed to greater social competence as resilient preschoolers transitioned into elementary school. These characteristics are similar to the protective factors associated with resilience found in other longitudinal studies in different populations.[6–8] It is important to highlight that these protective factors occurred naturalistically and retrospectively associated with resilience. Thus, the relevance and prospective applicability to prevention and early intervention are not self-evident. However, their relevance becomes more apparent when considered in the context of studies that have identified a relatively small set of antecedent risk factors that predict the development of a broad range of internalizing, externalizing problems, including substance use and other risky behaviors by adolescence. For example, early deficits in problem-solving skills in young children are associated with later development of depression, conduct disorder, and adolescent-onset substance use.[4,5] Poor behavioral and emotional regulation in young children has been shown to predict later development of anxiety, conduct problems, antisocial behavior, and substance abuse.[4,5] Similarly, preschool-aged children with social skills deficits that continue as they transition into elementary school are at increased risk of developing depression, social phobia, peer conflict, peer deviance, conduct disorders, delinquency, and substance abuse by adolescence.[4,5] This research underscores the importance of early childhood identification of emotional and behavioral dysregulation as well as deficits or delayed development of language and reading skills, problem-solving, and social skills. Early childhood deficits in these core skills increase the risk of developing development of a broad range of mental health and behavior problems, including substance abuse by adolescence. There is also encouraging evidence that interventions that specifically target or enhance these core skills may prevent or significantly reduce the risk of developing associated adverse outcomes, as discussed in the next section.

Common Elements of Evidence-Based Prevention Interventions

Of the hundreds of evidence-based substance prevention interventions, the vast majority are school-based programs that are rarely implemented in pediatric primary care or outpatient mental health settings. Clinicians and other child-care workers in non–school-based settings often have very limited, if any, training in evidence-based prevention interventions. Moreover, many school-based prevention programs are highly specific (eg, violence prevention, bullying prevention, pregnancy prevention, suicide prevention).[3–5] Schools and communities often have limited data to guide their selection of prevention programs to maximize reach with limited resources. To address this issue, 2 recent meta-analyses conducted by Boustani and colleagues[4,5] have focused on identifying "common practice elements" across evidence-based prevention interventions that can be used by a broad range of clinicians in various settings without the need for additional specialized training. Their meta-analysis of universal preschool and elementary school prevention programs identified the following 5 common elements across evidence-based prevention interventions: psychoeducation, problem-solving, communication skills, insight building, and social skills training.[4] In a separate review of adolescent universal prevention programs, 3 additional common practice elements were identified in prevention programs targeting older school-aged children and adolescents: cognitive coping strategies, self-esteem building, and self-monitoring/self-regulation skills.[5] It is striking, but perhaps not surprising, that the common elements of evidence-based prevention interventions generally target the same skills deficits included in the common core of antecedent risk factors that predict a range of adverse outcomes discussed previously. It is also striking, but perhaps not surprising, that longitudinal studies indicate that early childhood strengths in these core skills (ie, verbal/reading, emotional/behavioral regulation, social skills, problem-solving) seem to be protective and help resilient "at-risk" youth overcome adversities and achieve outcomes comparable to the outcomes of "low-risk" youths from stable and more advantaged families and home environments.[6–8] There are several federally sponsored evidence-based prevention programs that provide a multitude of excellent evidence-based in-home or community-based prevention services that are widely available and accessible, nationwide, to at-risk youth and families and/or infants and young children with developmental delays. Pediatric primary care clinicians play a critical role in linking youth and families to these important multicomponent federally sponsored prevention services which include the following:

Early Intervention Program for Infants and Toddlers with Disabilities (https://www2. ed.gov/programs/osepeip/index.html):a federally funded program through the US Department of Education available in all 50 states to children ages 0 to 2 years who are experiencing developmental delays in cognitive development, physical development, communication development, social or emotional development, or adaptive development.

- *Head Start/Early Head Start* (https://nhsa.org) is a federal program that partners with state childcare systems and agencies to promote school readiness of children from birth to age 5 years from low-income families by enhancing language skills and cognitive, social, and emotional development.
- *Child First* (https://www.childfirst.org) is a national, evidence-based, 2-generation model that works with very challenged "at-risk" families and children between the ages of 6 and 36 months. *Child First* provides intensive mental-health and home-visiting services focused on developing nurturing, consistent, and responsive parent-child relationships and connecting families to needed community-based services. In controlled trials, the *Child First* intervention has

been shown to have a large effect size on prevention or improving language and communication skills and reducing aggressive and defiant behaviors. Compared with "usual care," families receiving *Child First* services are nearly 39% less likely to be involved with child protective services and a 98% increase in access to community services and resources. Mothers who received the *Child First* Intervention were 64% less likely to suffer from depression or mental health problems compared with mothers in the "usual care" control group. *Child First* services for families and children exposed to violence show significant improvements in child social-emotional and behavioral health, decreased parental stress, and a greater than 80% increase in access to community-based services. *Child First* wraparound services also include the provision of mental health consultation for early childhood education/preschool programs. The intervention specifically targets preschool children with low protective factors and/or high behavioral problems. Controlled studies indicate that almost all children benefit from the *Child First* intervention, but those demonstrating lower resilience and greatest need benefit the most. In this subgroup, the *Child First* intervention demonstrated a large effect size (between 0.8 and 1.0) on increasing the number and strength of protective factors, initiative (ability to use independent thought and action to meet their needs), self-control (ability to experience and express a range of emotions in socially appropriate ways), attachment (development of relationships with significant adults), and behavioral concerns (challenging behaviors).[10]

One of the limitations of "common elements" prevention research to date is the lack of focus on family- or community-based targets of prevention interventions. Because only a subset of evidence-based prevention interventions includes family and/or community-based components, these elements are less likely to be identified in meta-analyses as common components across all prevention interventions. Here again, longitudinal studies of resilience may be informative about family and community protective factors. For example, in the Kauai Longitudinal Study, resilient children and adolescents were often involved in activities that developed special talents that gave them a sense of pride and enhanced self-efficacy and self-esteem. These activities also often facilitated further development of social skills by increasing interaction with peers and caring adult role models and mentors. Blueprints for Healthy Youth Development (https://www.blueprintsprograms.org/programs) provides further evidence of the protective effects of involving "at-risk" youth in such activities. Blueprints for Healthy Youth Development (Blueprints) is a registry of scientifically proven and scalable interventions that have been shown to prevent or reduce the likelihood of antisocial behavior, substance abuse, and promote healthy youth development. Many Blueprints prevention programs include practice elements that specifically target the core skills deficits discussed previously and others focus on family-risk factors. Some focus on enhancing protective factors using community-based resources that increase youth involvement in prosocial activities with peers and caring adult role models and mentors. For example, Big Brothers and Big Sisters of America is a well-known national mentoring program, recognized by Blueprints as a "certified promising program." The program matches a volunteer adult mentor to an at-risk child or adolescent (ages 6–18 years) to delay or reduce antisocial behaviors; avoid drugs and alcohol and other risky behaviors; improve academic success, attitudes, behaviors, peer and family relationships; strengthen self-confidence; and provide social and cultural enrichment. Most rural and urban communities in the United States have a variety of community-based resources (eg, community recreational centers) that provide opportunities for youth to be involved in a broad range of enjoyable prosocial activities

Table 1
Core skills deficits, "common practice elements," and protective/resilience promoting factors

Core Skills Deficits	"Common Practice Elements"	Protective/Resilience Promoting
	Psychoeducation	Involvement in prosocial activities that build self-esteem, self-efficacy, confidence
Verbal/language	Communication skills training	Involvement in activities that increase association with prosocial peers, adult role models, and mentors
Reading	Reading skills training	Parent/caregiver monitoring and behavioral management skills
Problem-solving skills	Problem-solving skills training	
Social skills	Social skills training	
Emotional/behavioral dysregulation	Cognitive coping strategies Self-monitoring skills	
	Insight building	
	Self-esteem building activities	

that foster the development of special talents, social skills, and relationships with peers and caring adult role models. Clinicians and others who work closely with children and adolescents would do well to identify local community resources with these characteristics within their communities. These resources can be leveraged as prevention resources to enhance protective factors by actively encouraging youth and family involvement.

Implications for Clinical Practice

The 3 lines of research discussed in this article—longitudinal studies, antecedent risk factors, and "common elements" research—provide convergent evidence that a relatively small group of core skills deficits in young children can be characterized as common antecedent risk factors for a broad range of internalizing and externalizing disorders, including substance abuse by adolescence. Early identification of these skills deficits in young children and interventions to bolster these skills could prevent or significantly mitigate the risk of developing substance use and a range of other mental health and behavior problems by adolescence. Most pediatric primary care clinicians and behavioral health clinicians in outpatient child/adolescent mental health settings routinely screen for developmental delays but lack specialized training in evidence-based prevention interventions. However, most behavioral health clinicians do have training and frequently use many of the "common elements" (listed in Table 1) of prevention interventions within the scope of their practice. Busy primary care clinicians have the training but lack sufficient time to deliver prevention interventions beyond brief screening, psychoeducation, or very brief interventions and most refer infants and children with developmental delays (Early Intervention Program for Infants and Toddlers with Disabilities) and "at-risk" youth and families (Child First) to one of the aforementioned federally sponsored prevention programs.

SUMMARY

Many schools, but few pediatric primary care and outpatient child/adolescent behavioral health treatment settings implement evidence-based prevention interventions that have been shown to reduce the risk of substance abuse and other adverse outcomes by adolescence. Clinicians in these settings routinely screen for developmental delays and other risk factors but often lack the training and/or the time to deliver evidence-based prevention interventions within their scope of practice. Pediatric primary care and outpatient child/adolescent behavioral health settings currently represent a large but underutilized prevention resource and clinical workforce in the United States In 2021, the US Surgeon General, Vivek Murthy, MD issued a national advisory, calling attention to the urgent need to address the mental health crisis among the nation's youth. The American Academy of Pediatrics, the American Academy of Child and Adolescent Psychiatry, and the Children's Hospital Association characterized the current youth mental health as a national emergency. The youth mental health crisis is further fueled and underpinned by a global pandemic and the ongoing opioid epidemic. There is also growing evidence that the youth mental health crisis is further exacerbated by the rapidly expanding legalized cannabis environment. An increasing number of our nation's youth (and their adult caretakers) are using high potency cannabis products that are widely available in legalized markets. Cannabis use during adolescence complicates the clinical management of preexisting mental health problems and significantly increases the risk of developing psychosis, suicidality, depression, and anxiety disorders in adolescents and young adults.[1,2]

We can no longer afford to underutilize any sector of the community or clinical workforce. The current youth mental health crisis calls for an "all-hands-on-deck" approach to prevention, early intervention, and treatment. The goal of this article is to provide clinicians and others who work with children and adolescents across all settings with research-based information to identify early childhood risk factors, practical clinical tools (ie, "common elements") to mitigate risk, and community-based prevention resources and services that are currently available to "at-risk" youth and families.

CLINICS CARE POINTS

- To identify early childhood emotional/behavioral dysregulation and delays in verbal/language, reading, problem-solving, and social skills development
- To be familiar with local, state, and federally-funded early childhood prevention and intervention resources & programs for youth and families
- To encourage parents/caregivers to encourage child involvement activities that enhance self-esteem, self-efficacy, and confidence and increase association with pro-social peers and adult role models
- Teach parents/caregivers developmentally appropriate behavioral management and monitoring skills

DISCLOSURE

This work was supported in part by a grant from the National Institute on Drug Abuse (R01 DA053288). The content is solely the responsibility of the author and does not necessarily represent the official views of the National Institutes of Health. The author has no other conflicts of interest to declare.

REFERENCES

1. National Institutes of Health, National Institute on Drug Abuse. Principles of substance abuse prevention for early childhood: a research-based guide. 2016.

Available at: https://nida.nih.gov/publications/principles-substance-abuse-prevention-early-childhood/table-contents. Accessed January 28, 2022.

2. Substance Abuse and Mental Health Services Administration (SAMHSA). Preventing Marijuana Use among youth. Rockville, MD: National mental health and substance Use Policy Laboratory. Substance abuse and mental health services Administration; 2021. SAMHSA Publication No. PEP21-06-01-001.

3. Catalano RF, Mazza JJ, Harachi TW, et al. Raising healthy children through enhancing social development in elementary school: results after 1.5 years. J Sch Psychol 2003;41(2):143–64.

4. Boustani MM, Frazier SL, Chu W, et al. Common elements of childhood universal mental health programming. Adm Policy Ment Health 2020;47(3):475–86.

5. Boustani MM, Frazier SL, Becker KD, et al. Common elements of adolescent prevention programs: minimizing burden while maximizing reach. Adm Policy Ment Health 2015;42(2):209–19.

6. Werner EE. What can we learn about resilience from large-scale longitudinal studies?. In: Goldstein S, Brooks R, editors. Handbook of resilience in children. Boston, MA: Springer; 2013. p. 87–102.

7. Werner EE. Resilience and recovery: findings from the Kauai longitudinal Study. FOCAL POiNT: research, Policy, and practice in Children's mental health. Summer 2005;19(1):11–4.

8. Cosco TD, Kaushal A, Hardy R, et al. Operationalising resilience in longitudinal studies: a systematic review of methodological approaches. J Epidemiol Community Health 2017;71(1):98–104.

9. Jaffee SR. Sensitive, stimulating caregiving predicts cognitive and behavioral resilience in neurodevelopmentally at-risk infants. Dev Psychopathol 2007;19(3): 631–47.

10. Crusto CA, Whitson ML, Feinn R, et al. Evaluation of a mental health consultation intervention in preschool settings. Best Pract Ment Health 2013;9(2):1–21.

Substance Use Screening, Brief Intervention, and Referral to Treatment in Pediatric Primary Care, School-Based Health Clinics, and Mental Health Clinics

Jessica B. Calihan, MD, MS[a,b,*], Sharon Levy, MD, MPH[b,c]

KEYWORDS

• Adolescent • Cannabis use • Screening • Brief intervention • Referral to treatment

KEY POINTS

• Addressing cannabis use is an important part of comprehensive adolescent care, particularly given the current prevalence of adolescent use, availability of new potent products, decreased risk perception associated with legalization, and potential adverse developmental effects.

• Screening, brief intervention, and referral to treatment can be effectively implemented in multiple settings with the support of provider training and available evidence-based treatment resources and technology.

• There is a need for new and improved evidence-based strategies for brief intervention and referral to treatment.

INTRODUCTION

Screening, brief intervention, and referral to treatment (SBIRT) is a comprehensive framework for identifying substance use and intervening to reduce use and consequences. SBIRT was initially promoted as an approach to reduce drinking in adults with alcohol-related medical consequences.[1] Subsequently, the approach was

This article originally appeared in *Child and Adolescent Psychiatric Clinics*, Volume 32 Issue 1, January 2023.
 a Division of Adolescent and Young Adult Medicine, Boston Children's Hospital, 300 Longwood Avenue, Boston, MA 02115, USA; b Division of Addiction Medicine, Boston Children's Hospital, 300 Longwood Avenue, Boston, MA 02115, USA; c Harvard Medical School, Boston, MA 02115, USA
* Corresponding author.
E-mail address: jessica.calihan@childrens.harvard.edu

Abbreviations	
CUD	Cannabis use disorder
MI	Motivational interviewing
SBIRT	Screening, brief intervention, and referral to treatment
SU	Substance use
SUD	Substance use disorder

adapted for use with adolescents, and in this context, SBIRT expanded to include primary prevention efforts aimed at delaying the onset of substance use (SU) in this age group.[2]

In 2011, the American Academy of Pediatrics (AAP) officially recommended SBIRT as part of routine medical care for adolescents and published guidance for health care providers on best practices.[2] Since that time, there have been efforts to develop accurate screening tools, effective brief interventions (BI), and, to a lesser extent, strategies for effectively referring teens to SU treatment programs. Despite these efforts, the most recent US Preventive Services Task Force (USPSTF) review of SBIRT in 2018 resulted in an "I" statement for adolescent screening and BI, indicating that the evidence base is currently insufficient to support this practice.[3] Nonetheless, based on promising studies and lack of evidence of harm, several professional organizations and government agencies continue to recommend adolescent SBIRT as part of routine medical care.[4–6] Furthermore, government agencies and private foundations have made substantial investment to improve SBIRT education, implementation, and dissemination.

Cannabis is the third most commonly used substance among adolescents and, when used in this developmentally vulnerable stage, has unique medical, psychiatric, and cognitive consequences.[7–13] The use of SBIRT to prevent, delay, or decrease adolescent use and associated risks is particularly important now given the sharp decline in perception of cannabis-associated risks with legalization of medical and recreational cannabis, availability of new and more potent forms of cannabis, and intensification of SU among at-risk adolescents during the COVID-19 pandemic.[7,14–18] It is therefore crucial that pediatric primary care, behavioral health, and school-based providers have the necessary screening tools, BI skills, and training to identify and effectively address problematic SU. This article provides an update on the evidence base for screening, BI, referral to treatment (RT), and the current state of implementation focused on management of cannabis use disorder (CUD).

The realities of adolescent cannabis use and related consequences highlight the need for effective, evidence-based screening and treatment. SBIRT is a useful framework for incorporating SU prevention and early intervention in general pediatrics practices, behavioral health clinics, emergency departments (ED), and schools (**Fig. 1**).

Health care settings may be an ideal place to implement SU screening, identify at-risk youth, promote protective factors, and provide BIs, as most adolescents see a provider at least annually.[19] Research suggests that adolescents are willing to discuss SU with their providers, and parents and adolescents recognize the benefits of SBIRT provided in primary care.[20,21] Access to a medical home has expanded since implementation of the Affordable Care Act with increases in primary care utilization by publicly insured, low-income, black, and Hispanic adolescents.[22] In primary care settings, SBIRT implementation with and without embedded behavioral health care practitioners is feasible and associated with decreased mental health diagnoses at 1-year follow-up, and decreased SU diagnoses and emergency department (ED) visits at 3-year follow-up post implementation.[23–26] Despite the potential of SBIRT, a national study found few pediatricians report implementing all SBIRT components.[27]

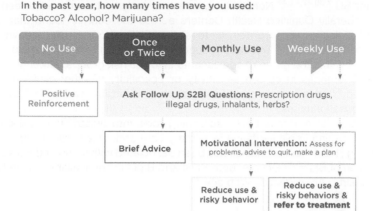

In the past year, how many times have you used:
Tobacco? Alcohol? Marijuana?

No Use	Once or Twice	Monthly Use	Weekly Use

Positive Reinforcement	Ask Follow Up S2BI Questions: Prescription drugs, illegal drugs, inhalants, herbs?

Brief Advice	Motivational Intervention: Assess for problems, advise to quit, make a plan

Reduce use & risky behavior	Reduce use & risky behaviors & refer to treatment

Fig. 1. S2BI algorithm. (© Boston Children's Hospital 2014. All rights reserved. This work is licensed under a Creative Commons Attribution-Non Commercial 4.0 International License.)

More than 50% of adolescents do not receive a well visit annually.[22] Given the need to address adolescent SU, there have been efforts to expand penetration of SBIRT to non-primary care settings, including subspecialty medical care, community mental health centers, EDs, and schools. A burgeoning body of research has found that SBIRT is feasible in community mental health settings,[28] can be provided effectively and at low cost in the ED,[29] and is more cost-effective than standard care for adolescents.[30] Universal SBIRT delivery in schools has the potential to reach large numbers of adolescents, and delivery of BI by school behavioral health counselors (BHC) or health educators is well-received by students and school nurses, promotes abstinence, and has been associated with decreased SU.[31–34]

SCREENING

The first step in SBIRT, screening, aims to define an adolescent's experience with SU and identify adolescents who are likely to have a disorder, in order to guide an appropriate intervention. Evidence suggests that screening with structured tools in pediatric primary care during well and acute care visits is feasible and practical for identifying youth with substance use disorders (SUD). Evidence-based structured screening tools that have been validated for use with adolescents include Screening to Brief Intervention (S2BI), Brief Screening Instrument for Adolescent Tobacco, Alcohol, and Drug Use (BSTAD), and Alcohol, Smoking, and Substance Involvement Screening Test (ASSIST).[35–37] These tools all screen for the most common substances used by teens: alcohol, nicotine, and cannabis, and either initially screen for additional substance categories (ASSIST) or prompt additional screening if an adolescent endorses any SU (S2BI, BSTAD). When a screen suggests high risk for an SUD, health care providers can follow up with CRAFFT (Car, Relax, Alone, Family, Forget, Trouble) questions, the GAIN questionnaire (Global Appraisal of Individual Needs), which assesses for SU and co-occurring mental health disorders, or perform an unstructured interview to probe about substance-related consequences to begin a discussion exploring potential targets for further motivational interviewing (MI).[38–40]

National surveys and research trials evaluating screening instruments consistently find higher rates of adolescent SU disclosure compared with clinical samples, thereby suggesting adolescents may be more comfortable with anonymous and confidential screens for SU.[7,36,37,41,42] Nonetheless, a recent study that examined screen results from 15 Federally Qualified Health Centers across the country found that rates of "high-risk" clinical screens were similar to rates of SUD reported in the anonymous national household survey.[42] This finding suggests that much of the nondisclosure may be occurring within the group of adolescents in lower-risk groups. Although there are not clear differences in screen sensitivity or specificity whether clinician- or self-administered,[43] adolescents report feeling more comfortable and honest completing electronic questionnaires.[44]

Incorporation of evidence-based screening tools into electronic medical records supports screening implementation in primary care and, when paired with brief provider training (1–2 1-hour sessions), has been associated with increased SU screening and provision of BIs.[25,45] Of note, both S2BI and BSTAD are available on the National Institute of Drug Abuse (NIDA) Web site.[46]

BRIEF INTERVENTION

The second step of SBIRT is patient-centered BI, or a provider-patient conversation focused on encouraging healthy choices to prevent, reduce, or stop SU and related risk-taking behaviors. The AAP recommends that health care providers educate patients about the potential cognitive, psychiatric, and physical harms of cannabis use and provide clear advice regarding abstinence or cessation.[6] Although there is no evidence that screening *increases* the risk of an adolescent using substances, teens who report no past year use can benefit from positive reinforcement with normative corrective statements emphasizing the true low prevalence of SU. For adolescents whose screen result indicates heightened risk for CUD, a discussion of the benefits and risks of substance-related consequences combined with clear advice to quit is recommended.[40]

BI can be performed by primary care providers or other members of the health care team. Engaging BHCs to provide BI may improve mental health in addition to SU outcomes.[25,26] However, many adolescents decline referral, making primary care providers more likely to deliver BI even in settings where MH providers are available.[45]

Several structured BIs have been developed and tested with youth in medical settings. In primary care, Peer Network Counseling, which consists of a 20-minute session administered by therapists,[47,48] and Project CHAT, which consists of a 15- to 20-minute MI intervention with a 5- to 10-minute reminder phone call administered by trained case managers,[49,50] have both been shown to decrease cannabis use and related consequences up to 12 months postintervention. In France, the FRAMES BI model, which consists of a physician-administered initial BI visit and 3 follow-up sessions over 12 months, was associated with decreased cannabis use 6 and 12 months' postintervention.[51] Project CHILL, which consists of 1 session with an MI-trained therapist or use of an animated, 30- to 40-minute interactive computer program, found that computerized BI was more effective at reducing adolescent cannabis use over 12-month follow-up compared with when similar content was delivered in-person.[52] The MOMENT intervention, comprising two 60-minute sessions with counselors and enhanced with mobile technology–facilitated self-monitoring and motivational messaging, was found to be acceptable to youth and effectively reduced cannabis cravings at 3-month follow-up.[53] Healthy Choices, which consists of four 60-minute sessions delivered by a trained therapist, was associated with decreased cannabis use at 15-month follow-up among adolescents with HIV who used cannabis less than 4 times weekly at baseline.[54] Youth presenting to the ED who received the Brief Negotiated Interview, which is administered by a trained health promotion advocate during an initial 20- to 30-minute session with a booster telephone call 10 days later, were found to have reduced cannabis use and related consequences than controls at 3- and 12-month follow-up.[55]

Studies of school-based SBIRT have found that students generally have positive attitudes toward school SBIRT programs[32]; it is feasible to recruit non-treatment-seeking adolescents for interventions with a school health educator,[56] and that interventions can reduce cannabis use and related consequences.[57]

A meta-analysis of 26 studies found that across various settings, BI implemented by clinicians or trained providers are effective at decreasing cannabis use and related consequences.[58]

REFERRAL TO TREATMENT

Adolescents with moderate to severe CUD with risk factors for severe substance-related consequences or who are unable to reduce cannabis use in response to BI may benefit from referral to specialty care for comprehensive evaluation and evidence-based treatment.[40] There are numerous psychosocial/behavioral substance treatment interventions with proven efficacy for SUD in adolescents and young adults as reviewed/discussed in more detail in *article 11* of this volume. The American Society of Addiction Medicine Criteria provide guidance about appropriate level of care based on an individual patient's needs, strengths, resources, supports, obstacles, and potential for risk or self-harm.[59]

RT is the least studied and often the least implemented aspect of SBIRT. Options for care are limited, as only a quarter of US addiction treatment facilities offer services for adolescents, and only 1% of all addiction medicine board-certified providers are pediatricians.[60] A recent study of SBIRT implemented in primary care clinics found only 4 of 165 adolescents with problematic SU were referred to specialty care,[45] and another study found that fewer than half of adolescents who received referrals to addiction specialty programs engaged in care.[28] Provider support and counseling may facilitate referral,[61] although there is a significant need for more evidence-based strategies to support adolescent engagement in treatment.[40]

Primary care–addiction medicine partnerships are a promising resource for provision of SU treatment in primary care and facilitating referrals for adolescents in need of more support.[62–64]

BARRIERS TO SCREENING, BRIEF INTERVENTION, AND REFERRAL TO TREATMENT IMPLEMENTATION

Logistical barriers to SBIRT implementation include clinic time limitations, insufficient staff and/or technology for screening, concerns regarding confidentiality, and lack of referral resources.[27,63,65] Although time is the most commonly reported barrier, this concern may be exaggerated. Clinician screening requires 74 seconds on average (62 seconds if no past-year use, 116 seconds if any past-year use), and self-administered electronic screens are even more time-efficient.[43] A survey in Massachusetts found that most adolescent-serving providers were able to provide brief advice (83%), counseling (67%), and RT (74%) in less than 5 minutes.[63] Succinct guidance can be very impactful, as even a brief (2–3 minute) conversation with a health care provider about the harms of SU has been shown to reduce adolescent use.[24]

Limited provider knowledge regarding SBIRT efficacy and SU treatment is also a barrier to SBIRT implementation. National surveys of heath care providers have found that limited familiarity with screening tools, lack of SU treatment knowledge, and insufficient addiction training are associated with decreased SBIRT implementation.[27,65] Provider education on SBIRT and referral resources can help providers improve their practices. For example, a trial of SBIRT implementation for adolescents found that pediatricians provided three 60-minute educational sessions on SBIRT were more likely to provide SU-focused BI and refer to specialty SU or mental health treatment compared with trained BHC and untrained pediatricians.[25] A Massachusetts SBIRT initiative that involved mailing all practicing pediatricians an adolescent SBIRT toolkit was associated with increased pediatrician report of SBIRT knowledge, SU screening with validated tools, and RT.[63,66] SBIRT education in residency may also be effective in influencing future practice. One initiative that combined didactic training with a skills-based session on the Brief Negotiation Interview for pediatric residents was associated with improved adherence to BI principles on standardized patient scenarios and continued use of BI in clinical practice.[67]

Several adolescent SBIRT and office-based treatment resources are available for providers, including Web sites from individual state and national programs, online toolkits, virtual screens, and a provider locator from the Substance Abuse and Mental

Table 1
Online resources for providers

Name	Web Site	Description
Youth SBIRT	https://www.ysbirt.org/	Provides information to equip primary care providers with resources and support to implement SBIRT in their practice
Adolescent SBIRT Toolkit for Providers	https://massclearinghouse.ehs.state.ma.us/PROG-BSAS-SBIRT/SA1099.html	The Massachusetts Department of Public Health sponsored creation of an SBIRT guide for providers using the S2BI screening tool
SAMHSA SBIRT	https://www.samhsa.gov/sbirt	Provides SBIRT information and resources, including a help line for local resources, reimbursement coding guidance, and training opportunities
NIDA Screening for SU in the Pediatric/ Adolescent Medicine Setting	https://nida.nih.gov/nidamed-medical-health-professionals/science-to-medicine/screening-substance-use/in-pediatric-adolescent-medicine-setting	Includes information about screening, including links to virtual BSTAD and S2BI, and guidance for next steps if a patient screens positive
Providers Clinical Support System	https://pcssnow.org/	Created by SAMHSA to train primary care providers in evidence-based prevention and treatment of opioid use disorders. Includes information for adolescent providers
SAMHSA Provider Locator	https://findtreatment.samhsa.gov/	Providers and/or families can use the provider locator to find local substance use treatment services and helpful information (ie, languages spoken, insurance, and so forth)

Health Services (SAMHSA) that can be used to find local treatment resources (**Table 1**). Expanding these resources and educational programs could be beneficial in addressing the knowledge gaps that ultimately limit treatment options for youth.

There also continues to be a significant need for evidence-based, effective BI to address positive screens in primary care settings. In 2018, a USPSTF review found there was insufficient evidence to recommend adolescent SBIRT.[3] Similarly, in 2020, the USPSTF gave primary care-based screening for adolescent SU an "I" recommendation, again highlighting a lack of evidence-based interventions to address positive screens.[68] There are few evidence-based BIs specifically validated to address cannabis use in primary care, and positive results are mostly limited to short-term effects.[69] There is a need to rigorously evaluate models demonstrated effective in local settings to establish feasibility and external validity.

SUMMARY

Through SBIRT implementation, adolescent-serving providers have a valuable opportunity to address adolescent cannabis use as a modifiable health behavior that contributes to the leading causes of morbidity and mortality among youth in the United States.[70] There has been significant work, primarily funded by SAMHSA, to promote SBIRT implementation and research over the last 2 decades.[66,71] This has facilitated increases in pediatrician screening, use of validated tools, and preventive messaging, as indicated by a 2014 national survey of pediatricians showing 88% screen annually for SU and 92% provide prevention messages in response to negative screens.[27,63,66]

Although SBIRT has been associated with modest short-term reductions in cannabis use, further research is needed on interventions that are effective in the longer-term, and that prevent or delay cannabis initiation.[72]

Strategies for addressing cannabis use are particularly critical now given the legalization of cannabis, which have been decreased risk perception, and availability of a wide variety of more attractive and more potent products.[17,18,73] Furthermore, the rapid expansion of telemedicine during the COVID-19 pandemic has opened up new opportunities for adolescent SBIRT and SU care.[74,75]

CLINICS CARE POINTS

- Cannabis use is common. Changes in available products and potency have increased the risk of physical, psychological, cognitive, and developmental adverse effects

- Screening, brief intervention, and referral to treatment can be effectively implemented in multiple settings, including primary care clinics, mental health treatment programs, emergency departments, and schools

- The use of validated screening tools is critical for evaluation of adolescent substance use. Although there are some brief intervention associated with modest, short-term effects on cannabis use, there is a need for new and improved evidence-based strategies

- Referral to treatment remains challenging given limited treatment resources and evidence-based best practices for transfer of care. Partnerships between primary care and addiction specialists can capacitate medical homes to provide substance use treatment and support referrals to higher levels of care for adolescents when necessary

- Screening, brief intervention, and referral to treatment implementation can be supported by incorporating electronic screening into the electronic health record, training providers on components of brief intervention, using available personnel or technology resources, and providing providers with resources for evidence-based treatment

DISCLOSURE

The authors have nothing to disclose.

REFERENCES

1. Babor TF, del Boca F, Bray JW. Screening, Brief Intervention and Referral to Treatment: implications of SAMHSA's SBIRT initiative for substance abuse policy and practice. Addiction 2017;112:110–7.
2. American Academy of Pediatrics Committee on Substance Abuse. Substance use screening, brief intervention, and referral to treatment for pediatricians [Policy Statement]. Pediatrics 2011;128(5). https://doi.org/10.1542/peds.2011-1754.
3. Curry SJ, Krist AH, Owens DK, et al. Screening and behavioral counseling interventions to reduce unhealthy alcohol use in adolescents and adults: US preventive services Task Force recommendation statement. JAMA - J Am Med Assoc 2018;320(18):1899–909.
4. Hagan JF, Shaw JS, Duncan PM. Bright futures: guidelines for health supervision of infants, children, and adolescents [pocket guide]. 4th edition. Elk Grove Village, IL: American Academy of Pediatrics; 2017.
5. Substance Abuse and Mental Health Services Administration. Screening, brief intervention, and referral to treatment (SBIRT). SAMHSA. Available at: https://www.samhsa.gov/sbirt. Accessed October 19, 2021.
6. American Academy of Pediatrics Committee on Substance Use and Prevention. Substance use screening, brief intervention, and referral to treatment [Policy Statement]. Pediatrics 2016;138(1). https://doi.org/10.1542/peds.2016-1210.
7. Johnston LD, Miech RA, O'Malley PM, et al. Monitoring the Future national survey results on drug use 1975-2020: Overview, key findings on adolescent drug use. Ann Arbor: Institute for Social Research, University of Michigan; 2021.
8. Levine A, Clemenza K, Rynn M, et al. Evidence for the risks and consequences of adolescent cannabis exposure. J Am Acad Child Adolesc Psychiatry 2017;56(3):214–25.
9. Jacobus J, Tapert S. Effects of cannabis on the adolescent brain. Curr Pharm Des 2014;20(13):2186–93.
10. Scott JC, Slomiak ST, Jones JD, et al. Association of cannabis with cognitive functioning in adolescents and young adults A systematic review and meta-analysis. JAMA Psychiatry 2018;75(6):585–95.
11. Meier MH, Caspi A, Ambler A, et al. Persistent cannabis users show neuropsychological decline from childhood to midlife. Proc Natl Acad Sci U S A 2012;109(40).
12. Gruber SA, Silveri MM, Dahlgren MK, et al. Why So Impulsive? White Matter alterations are associated with Impulsivity in chronic marijuana Smokers. Exp Clin Psychopharmacol 2011;19(3):231–42.
13. Becker MP, Collins PF, Schultz A, et al. Longitudinal changes in cognition in young adult cannabis users. J Clin Exp Neuropsychol 2018;40(6):529–43.
14. ElSohly MA, Mehmedic Z, Foster S, et al. Changes in cannabis potency over the last two decades (1995-2014) - analysis of current data in the United States. Biol Psychiatry 2016;79(7):613–9. Changes.
15. Romm KF, Patterson B, Crawford ND, et al. Changes in young adult substance use during COVID-19 as a function of ACEs, depression, prior substance use and resilience. Substance Abuse 2021. https://doi.org/10.1080/08897077.2021.1930629. Published online.

16. Dumas TM, Ellis W, Litt DM. What does adolescent substance use look like during the COVID-19 pandemic? Examining changes in frequency, Social contexts, and pandemic-related predictors. J Adolesc Health 2020;67:354–61.
17. Hines LA, Freeman TP, Gage SH, et al. Association of high-potency cannabis use with mental health and substance use in adolescence. JAMA Psychiatry 2020; 77(10):1044–51.
18. Carliner H, Brown QL, Sarvet AL, et al. Cannabis use, attitudes, and legal status in the U.S.: a review. Prev Med 2017;104:13–23.
19. Adams SH, Park MJ, Irwin CE. Adolescent and young adult preventive care: comparing national survey rates. Am J Prev Med 2015;49(2):238–47.
20. Yoast RA, Fleming M, Balch GI. Reactions to a concept for physician intervention in adolescent alcohol use. J Adolesc Health 2007;41(1):35–41.
21. Stern SA, Meredith LS, Gholson J, et al. Project CHAT: a brief motivational substance abuse intervention for teens in primary care. J Subst Abuse Treat 2007; 32(2):153–65.
22. Adams SH, Park MJ, Twietmeyer L, et al. Increasing delivery of preventive services to adolescents and young adults: does the preventive visit help? J Adolesc Health 2018;63(2):166–71.
23. Parthasarathy S, Kline-Simon AH, Jones A, et al. Three-year outcomes after brief treatment of substance use and mood symptoms. Pediatrics 2021;147(1). https://doi.org/10.1542/PEDS.2020-009191.
24. Harris SK, Csémy L, Sherritt L, et al. Computer-facilitated substance use screening and brief advice for teens in primary care: an International trial. Pediatrics 2012;129:1072–82. www.aappublications.org/news.
25. Sterling S, Kline-Simon AH, Satre DD, et al. Implementation of screening, brief intervention, and referral to treatment for adolescents in pediatric primary care a cluster randomized trial. JAMA Pediatr 2015;169(11):e153145.
26. Sterling S, Kline-Simon AH, Jones A, et al. Health care use over 3 years after adolescent SBIRT. Pediatrics 2019;143(5). https://doi.org/10.1542/peds.2018-2803.
27. Hammond CJ, Parhami I, Young AS, et al. Provider and practice characteristics and perceived barriers associated with different levels of adolescent SBIRT implementation among a national sample of US pediatricians. Clin Pediatr 2021; 60(9–10):418–26.
28. Stanhope V, Manuel JI, Jessell L, et al. Implementing SBIRT for adolescents within community mental health organizations: a mixed methods study. J Subst Abuse Treat 2018;90:38–46.
29. Barbosa C, Cowell A, Bray J, et al. The cost-effectiveness of alcohol screening, brief intervention, and referral to treatment (SBIRT) in emergency and outpatient medical settings. J Subst Abuse Treat 2015;53:1–8.
30. Neighbors CJ, Barnett NP, Rohsenow DJ, et al. Cost-Effectiveness of a motivational intervention for alcohol-involved youth in a hospital emergency department. J Stud Alcohol Drugs 2010;71(3):384–94.
31. Mitchell SG, Gryczynski J, Gonzales A, et al. Screening, brief intervention, and referral to treatment (SBIRT) for substance use in a school-based program: services and outcomes. Am J Addict 2012;21:S5–13.
32. Chadi N, Levy S, Wisk LE, et al. Student experience of school screening, brief intervention, and referral to treatment. J Sch Health 2020;90(6):431–8.
33. Lunstead J, Weitzman ER, Kaye D, et al. Screening and brief intervention in high schools: school nurses' practices and attitudes in Massachusetts. Substance Abuse 2017;38(3):257–60.

34. Maslowsky J, Whelan Capell J, Moberg DP, et al. Universal school-based imple-
    mentation of screening brief intervention and referral to treatment to reduce and
    prevent alcohol, marijuana, Tobacco, and other Drug use: process and feasibility.
    Substance Abuse: Res Treat 2017;11. https://doi.org/10.1177/1178221817746668.
35. Levy S, Weiss R, Sherritt L, et al. An electronic screen for triaging adolescent sub-
    stance use by risk level. JAMA Pediatr 2014;168(9):822–8.
36. Gryczynski J, Kelly SM, Mitchell SG, et al. Validation and performance of the
    alcohol, Smoking and substance Involvement screening test (ASSIST) among
    adolescent primary care patients. Addiction 2015;110(2):240–7.
37. Kelly SM, Gryczynski J, Mitchell SG, et al. Validity of brief screening instrument for
    adolescent tobacco, alcohol, and drug use. Pediatrics 2014;133(5):819–26.
38. Knight JR, Sherritt L, Shrier LA, et al. Validity of the CRAFFT substance abuse
    screening test among adolescent clinic patients. Arch Pediatr Adolesc Med
    2002;156(6):607–14.
39. Dennis ML, Chan YF, Funk RR. Development and validation of the GAIN Short
    Screener (GSS) for internalizing, externalizing and substance use disorders
    and crime/violence problems among adolescents and adults. Am J Addict
    2006;15(SUPPL. 1):s80–91.
40. Levy SJL, Williams JF. American Academy of pediatrics committee on substance
    use and prevention. Substance use screening, brief intervention, and referral to
    treatment [clinical report]. Pediatrics 2016;138(1). https://doi.org/10.1542/peds.
    2016-1211.
41. Substance Abuse and Mental Health Services Administration. Key Substance
    Use and Mental Health Indicators in the United States: Results from the 2020 Na-
    tional Survey on Drug Use and Health (HHS Publication No. PEP21-07-01-003,
    NSDUH Series H-56).; 2021.
42. Soberay A, DeSorrento L, Pietruszewski P, et al. Implementing adolescent SBIRT:
    findings from the FaCES project. Substance Abuse 2021;42(4):751–9.
43. Harris SK, Knight JR, van Hook S, et al. Adolescent substance use screening in
    primary care: validity of computer self-Administered versus clinician-
    Administered screening. Substance Abuse 2016;37(1):197–203.
44. Jasik CB, Berna M, Martin M, et al. Teen preferences for clinic-based behavior
    screens: who, where, when, and how? J Adolesc Health 2016;59:722–4.
45. Mitchell SG, Gryczynski J, Schwartz RP, et al. Adolescent SBIRT implementation:
    generalist vs. Specialist models of service delivery in primary care. J Subst
    Abuse Treat 2020;111:67–72.
46. National Institute on Drug Abuse. Screening tools for adolescent substance use.
    Available at: https://nida.nih.gov/nidamed-medical-health-professionals/screening-
    tools-resources/screening-tools-adolescent-substance-use. Accessed January 21,
    2022.
47. Mason M, Light J, Campbell L, et al. Peer Network counseling with urban adoles-
    cents: a randomized controlled trial with moderate substance users. J Subst
    Abuse Treat 2015;58:16–24.
48. Mason MJ, Sabo R, Zaharakis NM. Peer Network counseling as brief treatment for
    urban adolescent heavy cannabis users. J Stud Alcohol Drugs 2017;78:152–7.
49. D'Amico EJ, Miles JNV, Stern SA, et al. Brief motivational interviewing for teens at
    risk of substance use consequences: a randomized pilot study in a primary care
    clinic. J Subst Abuse Treat 2008;35(1):53–61.
50. D'Amico EJ, Parast L, Shadel WG, et al. Brief motivational interviewing interven-
    tion to reduce alcohol and marijuana use for at-risk adolescents in primary care.
    J Consult Clin Psychol 2018;86(9):775–86.

51. Laporte C, Vaillant-Roussel H, Pereira B, et al. Cannabis and young users—a brief intervention to reduce their consumption (CANABIC): a cluster randomized controlled trial in primary care. Ann Fam Med 2017;15(2):131–9.

52. Walton MA, Resko S, Barry KL, et al. A randomized controlled trial testing the efficacy of a brief cannabis universal prevention program among adolescents in primary care. Addiction 2014;109(5):786–97.

53. Shrier LA, Burke PJ, Kells M, et al. Pilot randomized trial of MOMENT, a motivational counseling-plus-ecological momentary intervention to reduce marijuana use in youth. mHealth 2018;4:29.

54. Murphy DA, Chen X, Naar-King S, et al. Alcohol and marijuana use outcomes in the healthy choices motivational interviewing intervention for HIV-positive youth. AIDS Patient Care and STDs 2012;26(2):95–100.

55. Bernstein E, Edwards E, Dorfman D, et al. Screening and brief intervention to reduce marijuana use among youth and young adults in a pediatric emergency department. Acad Emerg Med 2009;16:1174–85.

56. Walker DD, Roffman RA, Stephens RS, et al. Motivational enhancement therapy for adolescent marijuana users: a preliminary randomized controlled trial. J Consult Clin Psychol 2006;74(3):628–32.

57. Walker DD, Stephens R, Roffman R, et al. Randomized controlled trial of motivational enhancement therapy with nontreatment-seeking adolescent cannabis users: a further test of the teen marijuana check-up. Psychol Addict Behav 2011;25(3):474–84.

58. Halladay J, Scherer J, MacKillop J, et al. Brief interventions for cannabis use in emerging adults: a systematic review, meta-analysis, and evidence map. Drug and Alcohol Dependence 2019;204. https://doi.org/10.1016/j.drugalcdep.2019.107565.

59. American Society of Addiction Medicine. The ASAM Criteria. 2022. Available at: https://www.asam.org/asam-criteria. Accessed January 30, 2022.

60. Alinsky RH, Hadland SE, Matson PA, et al. Adolescent-serving addiction treatment facilities in the United States and the availability of medications for opioid use disorder. J Adolesc Health 2020;67(4):542–9.

61. Tait RJ, Hulse GK, Robertson SI. Effectiveness of a brief-intervention and continuity of care in enhancing attendance for treatment by adolescent substance users. Drug and Alcohol Dependence 2004;74(3):289–96.

62. Alinsky RH, Percy K, Adger H, et al. Substance use screening, brief intervention, and referral to treatment in pediatric practice: a quality Improvement project in the Maryland adolescent and young adult health collaborative Improvement and Innovation Network. Clin Pediatr 2020;59(4–5):429–35.

63. Levy S, Wiseblatt A, Straus JH, et al. Adolescent SBIRT practices among pediatricians in Massachusetts. J Addict Med 2020;14(2):145–9.

64. Levy S, Mountain-Ray S, Reynolds J, et al. A novel approach to treating adolescents with opioid use disorder in pediatric primary care. Substance Abuse 2018;39(2):173–81.

65. Palmer A, Karakus M, Mark T. Barriers faced by physicians in screening for substance use disorders among adolescents. Psychiatr Serv 2019;70(5):409–12.

66. Levy S, Ziemnik RE, Harris SK, et al. Screening adolescents for alcohol use: tracking practice trends of Massachusetts pediatricians. J Addict Med 2017;11(6):427–34.

67. Ryan SA, Martel S, Pantalon M, et al. Screening, brief intervention, and referral to treatment (SBIRT) for alcohol and other drug use among adolescents: evaluation of a pediatric residency curriculum. Substance Abuse 2012;33(3):251–60.

68. Krist AH, Davidson KW, Mangione CM, et al. Screening for unhealthy drug use: US preventive services Task Force recommendation statement. JAMA - J Am Med Assoc 2020;323(22):2301–9.
69. D'Amico EJ, Parast L, Osilla KC, et al. Understanding which teenagers benefit most from a brief primary care substance use intervention. Pediatrics 2019; 144(2). https://doi.org/10.1542/peds.2018-3014.
70. U.S. Department of Health & Human Services. Centers for disease control and prevention. National center for health Statistics: adolescent health. Available at: https://www.cdc.gov/nchs/fastats/adolescent-health.htm. Accessed January 19, 2022.
71. Harris SK, Herr-Zaya K, Weinstein Z, et al. Results of a statewide survey of adolescent substance use screening rates and practices in primary care. Substance Abuse 2012;33(4):321–6.
72. Tanner-Smith EE, Wilson SJ, Lipsey MW. The comparative effectiveness of outpatient treatment for adolescent substance abuse: a meta-analysis. J Subst Abuse Treat 2013;44(2):145–58.
73. ElSohly MA, Mehmedic Z, Foster S, et al. Changes in cannabis potency over the last 2 decades (1995-2014): analysis of current data in the United States. Biol Psychiatry 2016;79(7):613–9.
74. Uscher-Pines L, Sousa J, Raja P, et al. Treatment of opioid use disorder during COVID-19: experiences of clinicians transitioning to telemedicine. J Subst Abuse Treat 2020;118. https://doi.org/10.1016/j.jsat.2020.108124.
75. Levy S, Deister D, Fantegrossi J, et al. Virtual care in an outpatient subspecialty substance use disorder treatment program. J Addict Med 2021;16(2):e112–7. Publish Ahead Print.

Brief Interventions for Cannabis Using Adolescents

Ken C. Winters, PhD[a],*, Holly Waldron, PhD[a,b], Hyman Hops, PhD[a,b], Tim Ozechowski, PhD[a], Aleah Montano, BA[a,b]

KEYWORDS

- Adolescence • Cannabis use • Brief interventions
- Key phrases: use of brief interventions • To address adolescent cannabis use

KEY POINTS

- Brief interventions offer a promising approach to address adolescents who are users of cannabis.
- Core elements of brief interventions are motivational interviewing, decisional balance exercise, and goal setting.
- Using a brief intervention needs to include a plan for possible referral for more services.

INTRODUCTION

Cannabis continues to be the most commonly used substances after alcohol among adolescents. For example, based on the 2019 National Survey on Drug Use and Health among youth 12 to 17-year-old surveyed, 16%, 13%, and 7%, respectively, reported having used marijuana within their lifetime, within the past year and the past month.[1] Among youth seeking treatment at state-funded substance use treatment facilities younger than 20 years old, by far the most common primary substance reported at treatment admission is cannabis.[2]

The potential effects of cannabis use on the health of adolescents continue to receive research attention. For example, a recent international panel of cannabis researchers was convened to review the scientific literature on issue of the effects of cannabis use on health and to provide "lower risk cannabis use guidelines."[3] They provided several recommendations regarding nonmedical cannabis use for reducing health harms, with each recommendation accompanied by a rating of the strength of the evidence (conclusive, substantial, moderate, limited, or insufficient/none).

This article originally appeared in *Child and Adolescent Psychiatric Clinics*, Volume 32 Issue 1, January 2023.

[a] Oregon Research Institute, 3800 Sports Way, Springfield, Oregon 97403-2536, USA; [b] 500 Marquette Avenue, NW, Suite 1200, Albuquerque, NM 87102, USA
* Corresponding author. 1575 Northrop Street, Falcon Heights, MN 55108.
E-mail address: winte001@umn.edu

One recommendation noted that there is "no universally safe level of cannabis use" (conclusive level of evidence); an additional recommendation was that "any use of cannabis use should be delayed until after late adolescence, or the completion of puberty, to minimize development-related vulnerabilities for harm" (moderate level of evidence).[3] Another health-related issue pertaining to adolescent use of cannabis was the risk of developing a cannabis use disorder (CUD), which significantly increases if cannabis use is initiated during adolescence.[4,5]

Perceptions of Harm

Concerns about adolescent cannabis use have correlated with changing policies that may contribute to changes in availability and/or perceived risk of use.[6] To date, 19 US states have legalized cannabis for commercial production and sale to adults for recreational use, and these states plus an additional 18 allow use for medicinal purposes (www.learnaboutsam.org). An accompanying trend that bodes poorly on health is the dramatic increase in the potency of delta-9-tetrahydrocannabinol (THC) in cannabis products (www.learnaboutsam.org). Use of such high-potency products may accelerate risks of addiction, mental illness, and other negative health effects.[5]

In the past 10 years, in general, the perceived risk by adolescents of cannabis use has generally declined and overall cannabis use has increased among US students in 8th, 10th, and 12th grades.[7] These views include diminishing perceptions that marijuana use is harmful,[8] and increasing perceptions that marijuana is less harmful than alcohol.[9,10] Such perceptions may be influenced in the family when parents are using cannabis for medicinal purposes or the family is located in a state that permits legal recreational use by adults.[11]

Communicating to an adolescent science-based health impacts of cannabis use may fall on deaf ears. Yet, highlighting health effects that are pertinent and meaningful to an adolescent may enhance problem recognition and willingness to change. For example, several potential negative harms of cannabis use that are relevant to an adolescent include disruptions to ongoing brain development, increased risk of mental illness and suicidal thoughts and suicidal behavior, impairment to all learning and driving ability, increased risk of repeated and severe bouts of vomiting and an acute overdose reaction (psychotic-like thoughts).[6]

BRIEF INTERVENTIONS IN THE CONTINUUM OF SERVICES
Need for More Accessible Service Options

Psychological approaches to treat adolescent substance use, despite evidence of their effectiveness,[12] are underutilized. It is estimated that only 5% of adolescents who meet criteria for a substance use disorder receive specialized treatment.[7] Moreover, the service gap is likely larger for adolescents who use cannabis and present with mild-to-moderate level problems in many youth-serving health systems and settings, including pediatric clinics, acute emergency departments, school health clinics, juvenile justice, homeless shelters, and mental health clinics.[13] It is unfortunate that there exist so many of these "missed opportunities" during which youth get connected to a youth-serving setting but do not get screened for and, when appropriate, receive some type of intervention for cannabis use issues. There are many sources contributing to this gap: lack of commitment from program administrators or inadequate resources to implement behavior change resources; poor staff training to implement low-intensity counseling approaches; and minimal inclination by adolescents to want to make changes about their cannabis use.[13]

One health service delivery response to this problematic situation is in the general category of brief interventions (BIs). Now part of an integrated approach known as Screening, Brief Intervention, and Referral and Treatment, a BI provides a relatively rapid approach to discuss and negotiate a plan of action for substance use behavior change.[14]

Brief Intervention Models

There are many forms of BIs for use with adolescents. Some are limited to a few minutes of conversation, and some are relatively intensive and consist of two to three full counseling sessions.[15] All are organized around motivational interviewing skills,[16] which is a goal-oriented method of communication that seeks to strengthen an adolescent's motivation for and commitment to reduce or stop substance use by eliciting and exploring both the adolescent's internal interest to change and the external forces that are supporting change.

A leading form of a BI for youth is a Brief Negotiated Interview (BNI; https://www.bu.edu/bniart/sbirt-in-health-care/sbirt-brief-negotiated-interview-bni/). Whereas variants exist, the six common elements of a BNI model are summarized in **Box 1**: Brief Screening; Discuss Results; Decisional Balance Exercise; Triggers and Cravings; Readiness to Change Ruler; and Plan of Change. These elements are organized around motivational interviewing techniques and cognitive behavioral strategies, two psychosocial-based behavior change approaches common to all BIs.[15,17]

Outcome Studies for Cannabis Brief Interventions

Three types of adolescent BIs in the published literature are based on their substance target: alcohol-specific and nondrug-specific types, both of which dominant the literature,[19] and cannabis-specific, of which there are only two. An informative meta-analysis conducted by Tanner-Smith and colleagues[19] provides insights as to the incremental effects on cannabis outcomes by the two dominant models. The investigators identified 30 experimental and quasi-experimental published studies that reported the effects of BIs on alcohol and illicit drug use among youth. Some of those interventions ($n = 7$) only targeted alcohol but also examined outcomes for other drugs; others ($n = 23$) targeted both alcohol and other drugs and measured outcomes for both. Overall, the multi-targeted BIs were effective in reducing alcohol and illicit drugs, including cannabis. However, the BIs that targeted only alcohol had no

---

Box 1
Common Features of a Brief Negotiated Interview

1. Brief Screening: An adolescent-validated screening tool is administered.

2. Discuss Results: The youth's responses to the screening questions are discussed. Emphasis is on clarifying the history of situations common to the youth's substance use.

3. Decisional Balance Exercise: The youth's perceived benefits of using substances and what negative consequences have been experienced are discussed.

4. Triggers and Cravings: The internal and external triggers that elicit use in the adolescent are identified and discussed.

5. Readiness to Change Ruler: An exercise to determine how central or important changing is to the adolescent and how able or confident he or she feels about making changes.

6. Plan of Change: Develop goals for reducing or stopping use of substances; goal setting should be specific, meaningful, and realistic.

significant secondary effects on cannabis and other untargeted illicit drug use. These results were quite consistent across studies; the effects were negligible with respect to the presence/absence of several therapeutic intervention components, time until follow-up, intervention length, and average age of participants. **Table 1** provides a summary of the alcohol and cannabis outcome data (effect sizes) for the two types of BIs (alcohol-specific and multi-targeted).

Cannabis-Specific Brief Interventions

Bernstein and colleagues[19] developed a BI intended for adolescents and emerging young adults (14 to 21 years old) who reported recent cannabis use while receiving care at a pediatric emergency department. The program consists of a 15 to 20 minute session based on motivational interviewing administered by a peer educator, who conducts a 10-min follow-up booster phone call at 10 days post-enrollment. Peer educators received extensive training pertaining to research protocols, motivational interviewing, and other implementation procedures. Outcome data indicated that the BI showed significantly higher rates of cannabis abstinence and reductions in cannabis consumption at both the 3- and 12-month follow-up points compared with two control groups (assessment only and non-assessment).

Teen Marijuana Check-Up (TMCU) is a school-based motivational enhancement (MET)-focused BI developed by Walker and colleagues.[20,21] Students in the two-session TMCU program receive MET therapy that pairs motivational interviewing strategies with normative and other feedback pertaining to cannabis use. A recent version of TMCU includes three additional 15-minute motivational check-ins at 3-month intervals, with the aim of reinforcing gains and increasing motivation for change.[21] TMCU has been primarily studied in the context of a voluntary intervention offered to high school students who are regular cannabis users but are not seeking treatment.[21] The investigators found that this voluntary feature attracted students whose levels of cannabis use were comparable to adolescents receiving drug treatment for a CUD.[21] Several formal evaluations support the program's efficacy. Outcome data have consistently showed TMCU is associated with greater decreases in cannabis use relative to students in delayed intervention and educational control conditions.[20,21] Also, the program has been adapted for use as part of a multidimensional treatment program for youth with a CUD.[21] **Table 2** provides an overview of the two cannabis-specific BIs for adolescents.

ADJUSTMENTS TO BRIEF INTERVENTIONS WHEN ADDRESSING ADOLESCENT CANNABIS USE

The research literature on BIs for adolescent cannabis users, albeit limited, confirms that the use of MET and cognitive behavioral therapy (CBT) is advisable when

Table 1
Summary of meta-analysis outcome data comparing two types of brief interventions [19]

BI Type	Number of Studies	Number of Computed Effect Sizes	Mean Effect Size for Alcohol Outcomes	Mean Effect Size for Cannabis Outcomes
Alcohol-specific BI	7	54: alcohol 13: cannabis	0.20[a]	0.00
Multi-targeted BI	23	128: alcohol 58: cannabis	0.17[a]	0.15[a]

[a] $P < .05$.

Table 2
Overview of the two adolescent cannabis brief interventions

BI Program	Source	Program Features	Outcomes
Bernstein's Cannabis Brief Intervention	Bernstein et al,[19] 2009	20 min intervention, delivered by trained peer educators; focuses on motivational interviewing strategies, and includes suggestions offered for referrals to community resources and specialty drug treatment services; clients also receive a 5- to 10-min booster phone at day 10 to review progress with change plan and discuss referral issues	At 12-mo follow-up, BI participants were more significantly likely to be abstinent and, among non-abstainers, reported fewer cannabis use days compared with the assessment control group
Walker et al.'s *Marijuana Check-Up*	Walker et al,[20] 2011; Walker et al,[21] 2016	Two sessions; first session focuses on motivation interviewing; second session consists of normative feedback, review of risk and protective factors, how much money is spent on cannabis, and possible impact of cannabis use on life goals	Positive outcomes (reduced cannabis use and fewer negative consequences) maintained at 6-, 9-, 12-, and 15-mo post-BI, as compared with assessment only control group; mixed benefits from repeated check-in sessions

Adapted from Bernstein, E., Edwards, E., Dorfman, D., Heeren, T., Bliss, C., & Bernstein, J. (2009). Screening and brief intervention to reduce marijuana use among youth and young adults in a pediatric emergency department. Academy of Emergency Medicine, 16, 1174–1185.

addressing cannabis using youth. For example, the Bernstein program[19] and TMCU[20,21] are primarily based on MET/CBT approaches. In this light, the authors view the core elements of a BI described in **Box 1** as highly relevant when applying BIs for cannabis abuse. Yet, there are some cannabis-specific adjustments that merit attention, which are discussed as follows.

Potency Issue

As noted above, the THC potency of contemporary cannabis products has trended upwards in striking ways; concentrates can consist of potency levels as high as 80% to 90%. The use of cannabis products with higher THC concentration is linked with greater risk for developing a CUD as well as other negative health outcomes (eg, disrupt brain development; increase risk for psychosis).[22,23] However, it is often difficult to know how much THC is being inhaled or ingested by an adolescent user, making personal efforts to limit the use of high-potency products challenging. In those states with legalized sale of cannabis products for adults, packaging labels often provide weight-based measures rather than potency-based measures, which allow people to purchase a small amount of high-potency products, with potentially high levels of intoxicating effects.

During a BI, assessing the potency of cannabis products used and discussing the risk of using high-potency cannabis with the adolescent is advisable. This discussion can benefit from the counselor using reflective statements in the face of a youth who is expressing the viewpoint that using high-potency cannabis products is not harmful. For example:

Adolescent: "I am not going to waste my time with weak weed. I can handle what I am using."

Counselor: "You are saying that the weed you use is ok for you. I wonder about the negative effects if you keep using this high-potency weed. What are thoughts about this?"

The counselor strives to address the issue of potency by not directly challenging the adolescent but by reframing the issue about possible negative health effects if use of high-potency cannabis were to continue. The counselor will want to inquire about what type of cannabis products the adolescent uses; if concentrated, high-potency products are favored (eg, dabs, wax), it is advisable to offer information regarding their risk to health. Consider printing and distributing fact sheets about high-potency cannabis provided by the National Institute on Drug Abuse (https://www.drugabuse.gov/publications/drugfacts/marijuana).

Managing Ambivalence and Resistance by the Adolescent

It can be expected that a counselor will often face ambivalence and other signs of resistance to change by the adolescent. In the face of the country's pro-cannabis environment, it can be challenging for the BI counselor to raise the adolescent's awareness of the potential harm of cannabis use and to increase his or her motivation to reduce or abstain from use. Even though some adolescents may express some readiness to change, many are likely to express pushback to changing their cannabis use behavior at some point during the intervention, especially in the context of peer influences.[24]

Among counseling options in the face of resistance by an adolescent; we offer two general suggestions.

1. Use motivational interviewing skills to address oppositions to an idea, observation, or plan to change. Below are three strategies based on motivational interviewing technique[16]:
   - Reflection (acknowledging the adolescent's disagreement without causing defensiveness, but also getting a handle on the validity of the adolescent's sources of perceptions about health effects).

   "It sounds like you've thought a lot about this. Tell me where you are learning about cannabis."
   - Siding with the resistance and reframing (acknowledging the validity of the adolescent's perspective and offering a new meaning or interpretation).

   "It makes sense that you say you like the way using marijuana makes you feel. It may even be something you turn to as a way to avoid bad thoughts or feelings you have sometimes."
   - Emphasizing personal control (communicating to the adolescent that it is their decision whether or not to make a behavior change).

   "No one knows you better than you do. In the end, you are the one to decide how using marijuana fits for you."

2. Seek a more balanced view about cannabis use from the adolescent, by discussing common misperceptions held by youth. There are excellent resources from the research community to support the process of educating adolescents about cannabis use on health. We recommend the resource already noted provided by the National Institute on Drug Abuse (https://www.drugabuse.gov/publications/drugfacts/marijuana) as well as one from the Smart Approaches to

Marijuana (https://www.learnaboutsam.org/toolkit/). Options may include the following:

i. Driving ability is not impaired when high on cannabis.
ii. Cannabis use does not harm brain development.
iii. My mental health is improved by using cannabis.
iv. Vaping cannabis is a healthy alternative to smoking.

All of these statements are worded to reflect that cannabis use is not harmful or safe. Yet, each has another side to that declaration. Based on advice from several focus groups conducted by the senior author with adolescents in recovery from treatment from a CUD, the authors provide several examples of ways to talk about misconceptions and myths about cannabis use. Within a motivational interviewing framework, it is also advisable to follow each statement with a request for feedback from the adolescent (eg, "What are your thoughts about this?" "Have you heard about this topic before?").

i. "Being high on weed can make a user more distracted and impair reaction time when driving a car.
ii. "The adolescent brain is still developing during the teen years and weed can damage this development."
iii. "Using weed might give a person temporary relief from your anxiety but in the long run the risk increases of having bigger problems with anxiety." "The same with depression; the user can get temporary relief but many users find the depression gets worse and become more suicidal over time."
iv. "Vaping is not entirely harmless. Vaping is not inhaling water vapor. Damage to your lungs still occur from the aerosol-like chemicals from a cannabis vape pen."

REFERRAL TO TREATMENT

Both the outcome literature and clinical experience support the perspective that a BI is rarely a "one-time" behavior change counseling event.[6,15] As noted above, the general finding in the adolescent BI outcome literature is that abstinence is rare and continued heavy use is still relatively prevalent at post-BI follow-up.[15,18,25] This extant outcome literature aligns with the authors' view that a BI is best regarded as a momentum starter for change, with additional steps required for significant clinical progress by the client to occur. It is common for adolescents receiving a BI to meet criteria for a mild or moderate diagnostic and statistical manual, 5th edition (DSM-5) substance use disorder,[6,15] an indication that the adolescent's problem severity level is such that more counseling is needed than what is provided by a BI.

Thus, after a BI, cannabis-using adolescents may benefit from more services in the form of a referral for treatment (RT). A BI provider is in an opportunistic position to facilitate this follow-up process. The therapeutic relationship already established with the adolescent can promote the discussion with the teenager toward a mutual agreement about next steps. Also, the provider has insights about the youth's clinical picture and contextual situation (eg, what health insurance is available; what barriers and promoters of accessing additional services exist). With an RT comes provider responsibility to provide necessary clinical information to the referral agency or program, to follow-up if the youth made the referral appointment, and if the role of case manager is appropriate, to provide continuing support and advice to the adolescent over the course of his or her recovery.

The first consideration in determining if an RT is appropriate is signs of poor progress with the BI. Examples of clinical indicators that a progress is *not being made* are the following: weak commitment to make changes (eg, "I will think about making changes"); agreed-upon goals are vague (eg, "I will reduce my use some"); and ambivalence about soon receiving a check-up call by the provider (eg, "I am not so sure about that").

There are other factors when considering an RT: age of the adolescent, what risk and protective factors are present, and availability of adolescent-appropriate services.[6,15] Also, co-occurring mental or behavioral disorders (COMBDs) may have been found that require more services. There is a high prevalence of COMBDs among youth with cannabis use issues.[26,27] Whether the cannabis use preceded the COMBD or vice versa, clinical attention on any COMBD has merit. When ignored, progress with addressing the adolescent's cannabis use problem may be impeded.

An RT can take several forms[6,15]: a "warm handoff" to a specialty service within the provider's clinic, a referral to a local community agency (eg, a short-term or long-term outpatient or residential drug treatment program), and a decision for the BI provider to deliver booster counseling sessions or for a thorough clinical assessment.

If an RT is made, the provider must determine whether to involve parents in the referral decision and treatment planning. Many adolescents who seek care may request that their parents not be notified of their substance use and need for services,[28] yet some states require parental consent for an adolescent to receive drug treatment. Also, confidentiality cannot be preserved if the parents' health insurance will be paying for treatment. Clinical judgment is needed when weighing the pros and cons of breaking or maintaining confidentiality with the adolescent regarding this referral issue. Also, it can be expected that most adolescents who have received a BI are not going to readily accept an RT when indicated. A counselor wish to use the motivational interviewing strategies discussed earlier to deal with possible push back or resistance to change.

NEW DIRECTIONS

Extant BI models for youth are mostly fixed with respect to content and length, tend to be delivered in traditional fashion, and rarely (if at all) address co-occurring problems. The investigators view these limitations as missed opportunities to optimize the use of the BI approach for cannabis-using adolescents. Also, given the many challenges in motivating adolescents to make significant behavior changes, there is merit for the field to develop and test novel strategies. The authors highlight three promising directions that offer promise to enhance access and engagement and to improve outcomes.

Involving Parents in the Brief Intervention

The role of parents in adolescent BIs is underutilized. There is only one adolescent BI program in the research literature that formally includes significant parent involvement (*Teen Intervene*; 30, 31), yet such involvement was shown to add incremental benefits. In a comparison between a two-session adolescent only condition and a two-session adolescent plus a single parent session, the latter condition was associated with superior adolescent cannabis use outcomes at both 6- and 12-month follow-up.[29,30]

This general trend for adolescent BIs to not include parents is an example of a missed opportunity. Parents are in a unique position to help promote adolescent behavior change by virtue of their ongoing access to the teenager, multiple opportunities to provide continuous consistent messages, numerous teachable moments in real-world situations, and the opportunity to influence family norms and expectations.[31] Adolescents whose parents have used marijuana are about three times more likely to use cannabis than adolescents whose parents have never used cannabis,[32] and when parents do not believe cannabis use is harmful, or have permissive expectations about underage cannabis use, adolescents are more likely to use cannabis in comparison to adolescents whose parents have and express anti-cannabis attitudes.[33]

The prevention research literature,[31,32,34] as well as content from the *Teen Intervene* parent session,[29] provides a source of four topics to discuss if parents are participants in a BI program that addresses adolescent cannabis use:

1. Maintain the family policy that cannabis use during adolescence is not allowed
2. Avoid minimizing the potential harmful effects of cannabis use
3. (If relevant): Express regret about your own use of cannabis when an adolescent
4. (If relevant): Store your medicinal cannabis securely and avoid using it in the presence of the adolescent.

Technology-Based Interventions

Technology-based interventions (TBIs) represent a range of interventions that deliver treatment services either partially or entirely via computer, web, or mobile devices.[35,36] This type of low-cost, youth-centered resource may be particularly adolescent-friendly, which will enhance intervention engagement and fidelity.[37] Features include animated simulations, automated and daily feedback, video testimonies by youth, and other technology-based features.

Research by Walton and colleagues[38,39] and a meta-analysis of TBIs[37] suggest that TBIs so far are associated with promising but mixed results when applied to cannabis-using adolescents. One example of a successful program for college students is the resource developed and tested by Riggs and colleagues.[36] They investigated a web-based intervention with heavy cannabis-using college students ($N = 298$). The intervention incorporated protective behavioral strategies for avoiding cannabis use with personalized feedback. Compared with an education-focused control group, the TBI condition was associated with reductions in self-reported cannabis use and an increase in use of protective behavioral strategies at 6-week follow-up. As noted in the Beneria and colleagues' meta-analysis,[37] the promise of TBIs to treat cannabis using adolescents will need to be put to the test with more research.

Personalized Interventions

Personalization models, including adaptive, sequential-adaptive, person-centered, coordinated design, sequential multiple assignment randomized trial(SMART), and other models, have been described in the literature.[40,41] Mostly used in medicine,[40] these approaches are beginning to emerge in the adolescent behavioral health arena to promote client-centeredness and improve outcomes. A personalized prescriptive approach offers a promising approach to effectively address causal heterogeneity and response variability compared with fixed-type interventions.[42,43] Also, this perspective is consistent with developmental theory highlighting adolescence as a period during which they are trying to find their own footings in a rapidly changing physical and physiologic environment. A youth-centered, individualized approach enables the adolescent to make several choices in terms of the type, order, and amount of content in which to engage, all serving to increase their own involvement and motivation to succeed. Promising signs that personalizing content boosts outcomes have been reported with respect to adolescent substance use[44,45] and with COMBDs, such as depression, anxiety, and weight control, are documented.[43]

The growth of individualized approaches can be enabled by technology delivered interventions (TDI) given the ease to which content and implementation features can be personalized with online or web-based intervention programs. Future research has the opportunity to see if the effectiveness of TDIs is enhanced when personalization features are central to the resource.

SUMMARY AND RESEARCH NEEDS

The BI model holds promise as an effective approach that will expand the reach of services to adolescents who have cannabis use-related problems. Strengths of BIs are their user-friendly approach as behavior change strategy with potential for application to a wide range of help-serving professionals of varying educational backgrounds. They can be readily implemented, within traditional counseling or computer-assisted formats,[46] across pediatric clinics, mental health programs, school health clinics, and juvenile justice diversion programs. There are evidenced-based BI models for adolescents that comprise a 10-min conversation as well as examples that include two to three sessions.[15] Yet, the modest outcomes from a BI in terms of cannabis abstinence or reductions in level of use give pause as to their value as a one-time, stand-alone counseling event.[25] The authors notice BIs for cannabis using adolescents as a first step in a process to initiate behavior change momentum, with the expectation that a BI facilitates a path forward for additional clinical assessment and/or treatment services.

The research needs for this relatively nascent field are numerous: how to best define outcome for a BI (eg, abstinence vs harm reduction goals); assessing outcomes with more racially and ethnically diverse adolescents than has been studied to date; identifying specific mechanisms of change (eg, role of parents after the BI); role of moderators in outcome (eg, social determinants of health); and testing algorithms to assist with clinical decision-making regarding the need for and type of post-BI services. Also, the next generation of BIs will benefit from technology components that will further the reach of services and provide options for highly personalized content and formats, particularly with respect to individualizing content for co-occurring problems.

DISCLOSURE

Partial support for the preparation of this manuscript provided by grant DA049070 from the National Institute on Drug Abuse. There are no commercial or financial conflicts of interest to disclose.

CLINICS CARE POINTS

- Brief interventions are best indicated for an adolescent whose use of cannabis is at a mild or moderate level (eg, less than daily use; no signs of loss of control).
- Skills in the use of motivational interviewing are necessary for effective implementation of a brief intervention.
- Referring an adolescent for additional services includes several options depending on the youth's progress with the brief intervention, motivation for more counseling, and availability of services.

REFERENCES

1. Center for Behavioral Health Statistics and Quality. Results from the 2019 National Survey on drug Use and health: Detailed tables. 2020. Available at: https://www.

samhsa.gov/data/sites/default/files/reports/rpt29394/NSDUHDetailedTabs2019/ NSDUHDetailedTabs2019. pdf.

2. Hasin DS, Kerridge BT, Saha TD, et al. Prevalence and correlates of DSM-5 cannabis use disorder, 2012-2013: Findings from the National Epidemiologic Survey on alcohol and related conditions-III. Am J Psychiatry 2016;173:588–99.

3. Fischer B, Robinson T, Bullen C, et al. Lower-Risk Cannabis Use Guidelines (LRCUG) for reducing health harms from non-medical cannabis use: a comprehensive evidence and recommendations update. Int J Drug Policy 2021. https://doi.org/10.1016/j.drugpo.2021.103381.

4. Volkow ND, Han B, Einstein EB, et al. Prevalence of substance use disorders by time since first substance use among young people in the US. (2021). JAMA Pediatr 2021;175:640–3.

5. Volkow ND, Swanson JM, Evins AE, et al. Effects of cannabis use on human behavior, including cognition, motivation, and psychosis: a review. JAMA Psychiatry 2016;73:292–7.

6. Hassan A, Harris SK, Knight JR. Primary care and pediatric se1tting: screening, brief intervention and referral to treatment (SBIRT). In: Kaminer Y, Winters KC, editors. Clinical manual of adolescent addictive disorders. 2nd edition. Washington, D.C: American Psychiatric Association; 2019. p. 75–96.

7. Substance Abuse and Mental Health Services Administration (SAMHSA). Preventing marijuana Use among youth. Rockville, MD: National Mental Health and Substance Use Policy Laboratory. Substance Abuse and Mental Health Services Administration; 2021. SAMHSA Publication No. PEP21-06-01-001.

8. National Institute on Drug Abuse. Marijuana drug facts. 2019. Available at: https://www.drugabuse.gov/publications/drugfacts/marijuana.

9. Mikos RA, Kam CD. Has the "M" word been framed? Marijuana, cannabis, and public opinion. PLoS One 2019;14. https://doi.org/10.1371/journal.pone.0224289.

10. National Academies of Sciences, Engineering, and medicine. The health effects of cannabis and cannabinoids: the current state of evidence and recommendations for research. Washington DC: National Academies Press; 2017. https://doi.org/10.17226/24625.

11. Dilley JA, Richardson SM, Kilmer B, et al. Prevalence of cannabis use in youths after legalization in Washington state. JAMA Pediatr 2019;173:192–3.

12. Waldron HB, Turner CW. Evidence-based psychosocial treatments for adolescent substance abuse. J Clin Child Adolesc Psychol 2008;37:238–61.

13. Winters KC, Mader J, Budney AJ, et al. Interventions for cannabis use disorder. Curr Opin Psychol 2021;38:67–74.

14. Ozechowski TJ, Becker SJ, Hogue A. SBIRT-A: Adapting SBIRT to maximize developmental fit for adolescents in primary care. J Substance Abuse Treat 2016;62:28–37.

15. Winters KC. Adolescent brief interventions. J Drug Abuse 2016;2:1–3.

16. Miller WR, Rollnick S. Motivational interviewing: Helping people change. NY: Guilford press; 2012.

17. Sabioni P, Le Foll B. Psychosocial and pharmacological interventions for the treatment of cannabis use disorder. F1000Research 2018. https://doi.org/10.12688/f1000research.11191.1.

18. Tanner-Smith EE, Steinka-Fry KT, Hennessy EA, et al. Can brief alcohol interventions for youth also address concurrent illicit drug use? Results from a meta-analysis. J Youth Adolescence 2015;44:1011–23.

19. Bernstein E, Edwards E, Dorfman D, et al. Screening and brief intervention to reduce marijuana use among youth and young adults in a pediatric emergency department. Acad Emerg Med 2009;16:1174–85.
20. Walker DD, Stephens R, Roffman R, et al. Randomized controlled trial of motivational enhancement therapy with nontreatment-seeking adolescent cannabis users: a further test of the teen marijuana check-up. Psychol Addict Behaviors 2011;25:474–84.
21. Walker DD, Stephens RS, Blevins CE, et al. Augmenting brief interventions for adolescent marijuana users: the impact of motivational check-ins. J Consulting Clin Psychol 2016;84:983–92.
22. Di Forti M, Quattrone D, Freeman TP, et al. The contribution of cannabis use to variation in the incidence of psychotic disorder across Europe (EU- GEI): a multi-centre case-control study. Lancet Psychiatry 2019;6:427–36.
23. Van der Pol P, Liebregts N, Brunt T, et al. Cross-sectional and prospective relation of cannabis potency, dosing and smoking behaviour with cannabis dependence: an ecological study. Addiction 2014;109:1101–9.
24. Andrews JA, Hops H. The influence of peers on substance use. In: Scheier LM, editor. Handbook of drug Use Etiology. Washington, DC: American Psychological Association; 2010. p. 403–20.
25. Jensen CD, Cushing CC, Aylward BS, et al. Effectiveness of motivational interviewing interventions for adolescent substance use behavior change: a meta-analytic review. J Consulting Clin Psychol 2011;79:433–40.
26. Kaminer Y, Zajac K, Winters KC. Assessment and treatment of internalizing disorders (depression, anxiety disorders and PTSD). In: Kaminer Y, Winters KC, editors. Clinical manual of adolescent addictive disorders. 2nd edition. Washington, D.C.: American Psychiatric Association; 2019. p. 375–412.
27. Substance Abuse and Mental Health Services Administration (SAMHSA). Treatment considerations for youth and young Adults with serious emotional disturbances/serious mental illnesses and co-occurring substance use. Rockville, MD: National Mental Health and Substance Use Policy Laboratory, Substance Abuse and Mental Health Services Administration; 2021. Publication No. PEP20-06-02-001.
28. Reddy DM, Fleming R, Swain C. Effect of mandatory parental notification on adolescent girls' use of sexual health care services. JAMA 2002;288:710–4.
29. Winters KC, Fahnhorst T, Botzet A, et al. Brief intervention for drug abusing adolescents in a school setting: outcomes and mediating factors. J Substance Abuse Treat 2012;42:279–88.
30. Winters KC, Lee S, Botzet A, et al. One-year outcomes of a brief intervention for drug abusing adolescents. Psychol Addict Behaviors 2014;28:464–74.
31. Rusby JC, Light JM, Crowley R, et al. Influence of parent–youth relationship, parental monitoring, and parent substance use on adolescent substance use onset. J Fam Psychol 2018;32:310–20.
32. Brook JS, Brook DW, Arencibia-Mireles O, et al. Risk factors for adolescent marijuana use across cultures and across time. The J Genet Psychol 2001;162: 357–74.
33. Vermeulen-Smit E, Verdurmen J, Engels R, et al. The role of general parenting and cannabis-specific parenting practices in adolescent cannabis and other illicit drug use. Drug and Alcohol Dependence 2015;147:222–8.
34. Hops H, Andrews JA, Duncan SC, et al. Adolescent drug use development. In: Handbook of developmental psychopathology. Boston, MA: Springer; 2000. p. 589–605.

35. Marsch LA, Carroll KM, Kiluk BD. Technology-based interventions for the treatment and recovery management of substance use disorders: a JSAT special issue. J Substance Abuse Treat 2014;46:1–4.
36. Riggs NR, Conner BT, Parnes JE, et al. Marijuana eCHECKUPTO GO: effects of a personalized feedback plus protective behavioral strategies intervention for heavy marijuana-using college students. Drug and Alcohol Dependence 2018; 190:13–9.
37. Beneria A, Santesteban-Echarri O, Daigre C, et al. Online interventions for cannabis use among adolescents and young adults: Systematic review and meta-analysis. Early Intervention in Psychiatry 2021. https://doi.org/10.1111/eip.13226.
38. Walton MA, Bohnert K, Resko S, et al. Computer and therapist based brief interventions among cannabis-using adolescents presenting to primary care: one year outcomes. Drug and Alcohol Dependence 2013;132:646–53.
39. Walton MA, Resko S, Barry KL, et al. A randomized controlled trial testing the efficacy of a brief cannabis universal prevention program among adolescents in primary care. Addiction 2014;109:786–97.
40. August GJ, Gewirtz A, Realmuto GM. Moving the field of prevention from science to service: Integrating evidence-based preventive interventions into community practice through adapted and adaptive models. Appl Prev Psychol 2010;14: 72–85.
41. Wolff JC, Garcia A, Kelly LM, et al. Feasibility of decision rule-based treatment of comorbid youth: a pilot randomized control trial. Behav Res Ther 2020;131. https://doi.org/10.1016/j.brat.2020.103625.
42. Murphy SA, Lynch KG, Oslin D, et al. Developing adaptive treatment strategies in substance abuse research. Drug and Alcohol Dependence 2007;88:S24–30.
43. Ng MY, Weisz JR. Annual research review: Building a science of personalized intervention for youth mental health. J Child Psychol Psychiatry 2016;57:216–36.
44. Braciszewski JM, Wernette GKT, Moore RS, et al. A pilot randomized controlled trial of a technology-based substance use intervention for youth exiting foster care. Child Youth Serv Rev 2018;94:466–76.
45. Conrod PJ. Personality-targeted interventions for substance use and misuse. Curr Addict Rep 2016;3:426–36.
46. Knight JR, Kuzubova K, Csemy L, et al. Computer-facilitated screening and brief advice to reduce adolescents' heavy episodic drinking: a study in two countries. J Adolesc Health 2018;62:118e20.

Treatment of Adolescent Cannabis Use Disorders

Zachary W. Adams, PhD[a],*, Brigid R. Marriott, PhD[a], Leslie A. Hulvershorn, MD[b], Jesse D. Hinckley, MD, PhD[c]

KEYWORDS

- Cannabis • Marijuana • Adolescents • Treatment • Psychotherapy
- Pharmacotherapy

KEY POINTS

- Individual and family-based psychotherapy and behavioral interventions, such as CBT, have the strongest evidence for treatment of adolescents with cannabis use disorder.
- N-acetylcysteine (NAC) has been shown to be effective in promoting abstinence during treatment.
- Although few medications for cannabis use disorder have been tested in adolescents, several promising candidates warrant further research.

INTRODUCTION

Cannabis use is common among adolescents with roughly 40% of US youth reporting any lifetime cannabis use and 15% reporting at least 1 sustained episode (1 + month) of daily cannabis use by 12th grade.[1] Roughly 4% of US youth aged 12 to 17 years met criteria in the last year for a cannabis use disorder (CUD).[2] Treating CUDs in adolescence may mitigate short- and long-term disruptions to social, academic, health, and cognitive functioning.[3,4] This review summarizes the literature on treatments shown to reduce cannabis use and/or CUD symptoms in youth (**Table 1**). Emphasis was placed on treatments evaluated in randomized controlled trials (RCTs) with cannabis-specific outcomes. The strongest evidence is for cognitive behavioral psychotherapies, which typically intervene upon factors that maintain cannabis use

This article originally appeared in *Child and Adolescent Psychiatric Clinics*, Volume 32 Issue 1, January 2023.

[a] Department of Psychiatry, Indiana University School of Medicine, 410 West 10th Street, Suite 2000, Indianapolis, IN 46202, USA; [b] Department of Psychiatry, Indiana University School of Medicine, 1002 Wishard Boulevard, Suite 4110, Indianapolis, IN 46202, USA; [c] Department of Psychiatry, University of Colorado School of Medicine, 13001 East 17th Place, MS-F546, Aurora, CO 80045, USA

* Corresponding author.

E-mail address: zwadams@iu.edu

Twitter: @DrZacharyAdams (Z.W.A.); @JHinckleyMDPhD (J.D.H.)

Psychiatr Clin N Am 46 (2023) 775–788
https://doi.org/10.1016/j.psc.2023.03.004
0193-953X/23/© 2023 Elsevier Inc. All rights reserved.

Table 1
Evidence-based psychotherapy and pharmacotherapy treatments for adolescent cannabis use disorder

Individual-Focused Therapies	Description
A-CRA	An individual-focused intervention that aims to increase an adolescent's engagement in their community and activities that are incompatible with substance use to reinforce and support recovery. Consists of weekly sessions over 12–14 wk that include 10 adolescent, 2 caregiver, and 2 family sessions and case management
CBT	An individual-focused, structured approach that concentrates on identifying patterns of substance use and learning and applying skills and strategies to reduce use. Treatment typically entails 12–20 weekly sessions
CM	Behavioral intervention typically delivered as an adjunct component along with other evidence-based interventions (ie, MET/CBT) in which rewards are provided for positive behaviors (eg, abstinence, attendance). Delivery of CM with adolescents includes clinic-delivered and/or caregiver-delivered CM, and CM methods include the Fishbowl method, voucher method, or point-and-level system
MET/CBT	An individual-focused intervention that combines CBT and MET, which involves the use of motivational interviewing to resolve ambivalence and increase motivation to reduce substance use. Treatment ranges from 5 to 12 weekly sessions in individual and/or group formats

Family-Based Therapies	Description
BSFT	Family-based intervention that focuses on improving family functioning to reduce adolescent substance use and other problems. Consists of 12–16 family sessions with services delivered in the home, clinic, and other community settings
FFT	Family-based intervention that entails modifying maladaptive family patterns and cognitive behavioral techniques. Treatment includes around 12–14 weekly sessions that can be delivered in the clinic or home
Family-based I-CBT	Family-based, integrated intervention for co-occurring substance use disorder and suicidality. Treatment includes adolescent, caregiver, and family sessions. Session delivery and length vary depending on adolescent clinical presentation and insurance
MDFT	Family-based intervention that focuses on 4 treatment domains: adolescent, parent, family environment and relationships, and extrafamilial. Sessions are conducted 1 to 3 times per week over 3–6 mo and include adolescent, caregiver, and family sessions
MST	Family-based intervention in which individual, family, peers, school, and community factors are addressed to reduce adolescent substance use. Treatment is intensive with sessions delivered one to several times per week in home and community settings across 3–5 mo and therapists available 24/7 to families
RRFT	An integrative treatment that addresses co-occurring trauma-related symptoms and risk behaviors (eg, substance use, risky sexual behavior). Treatment includes 16–20 weekly individual sessions with caregiver and family sessions conducted as needed

Pharmacotherapies[a]	Description
NAC	A well-tolerated antioxidant derived from L-cysteine used in combination with other therapeutic interventions to reduce cravings and withdrawal symptoms

Abbreviations: A-CRA, adolescent community reinforcement approach; BSFT, brief strategic family therapy; CBT, cognitive behavioral therapy; CM, contingency management; CUD, cannabis use disorder; FDA, US Food and Drug Administration; FFT, functional family therapy; I-CBT, integrated CBT intervention; MDFT, multidimensional family therapy; MET/CBT, motivational enhancement therapy/cognitive behavioral therapy; MST, multisystemic therapy; NAC, N-acetylcysteine; RRFT, risk reduction through family therapy.

[a] There are currently no FDA-approved pharmacotherapies for CUD in adolescents.

both external (eg, parental monitoring, rules, peer use) or internal (eg, expectancies, coping skills, cravings, motivation for change) to the adolescent.[4,5] The literature on pharmacotherapies for youth with CUD is also reviewed, because some medications may alleviate cannabis craving and withdrawal symptoms, facilitating reductions in cannabis use.[6,7] The article concludes by highlighting avenues for future CUD treatment research.

PSYCHOTHERAPIES FOR CANNABIS USE DISORDER IN ADOLESCENTS
Family-Based Therapies

Family-based interventions, which target the family system in addition to adolescent- and community-level factors, are considered well-established approaches to treating adolescent substance use.[8] A meta-analysis examining the comparative effectiveness of outpatient treatments for adolescent substance use found family-based therapies to be most effective.[9] Four such therapies are summarized that have been evaluated in at least 1 RCT in which cannabis-specific outcomes were reported.

Multidimensional family therapy

Multidimensional family therapy (MDFT) encompasses 4 treatment domains: adolescent (eg, coping, emotion regulation; alternative behaviors), parent (eg, parenting skills, involvement with adolescent), interactional (eg, family conflict, communication skills), and extrafamilial (eg, family competency in adolescent's social systems).[10,11] MDFT demonstrated reductions in cannabis use frequency across several RCTs.[11–16] For example, 1 study found a 20.1-day reduction in cannabis use days in the 90 days before a 12-month follow-up in the MDFT condition and 14.9-day reduction in the CBT condition.[16] Self-reported minimal use/abstinence rates ranged from 18.2% to 64% for adolescents who received MDFT across studies (vs 14.8%–44% in comparison conditions).[11,12,16] Another study examined substance use disorder (SUD) diagnosis at 12-month follow-up and found that 18% of adolescents who received MDFT no longer met criteria for a CUD (vs 15% in the comparison group), 38% of MDFT adolescents met criteria for cannabis dependence (vs 82% at baseline, 52% in the comparison condition), and 33% met criteria for cannabis abuse (vs 22% in the comparison group).[15] In 4 RCTs,[11,13–15] MDFT demonstrated greater or more rapid improvement in cannabis outcomes than the comparison conditions (ie, adolescent group therapy, multifamily education intervention, individual CBT, individual psychotherapy, peer group therapy), with small-medium to large effect sizes observed across studies.

Brief strategic family therapy

BSFT posits that reducing maladaptive interactions and increasing the family's use of more adaptive interactional patterns will reduce an adolescent's symptoms, including substance use.[17] In an RCT comparing BSFT to an adolescent-only group treatment,[18] a significant decrease in cannabis use was found for BSFT (41% no longer using at termination) compared with control (13%). Robbins and colleagues (2011)[19] compared BSFT with usual care in community-based adolescent outpatient drug abuse programs (where two-thirds of youth met criteria for CUD at baseline) and found no differences between the 2 conditions in substance use. A long-term follow-up of this study revealed no differences in cannabis or other substance use between treatments 3 to 7 years later.[20]

Multisystemic therapy

Multisystemic therapy (MST) leverages protective factors and targets risk factors across multiple levels of a youth's ecology to reduce substance use.[21] In an RCT comparing MST with usual community services, juvenile offenders reported a significant reduction in self-reported cannabis and alcohol use at posttreatment, but this reduction was not maintained at the 6-month follow-up and no significant between-group treatment effects were found.[22] A 4-year follow-up of this RCT revealed no significant change in self-reported substance use; however, those who had been in the MST condition had significantly higher rates of cannabis abstinence (55%) than those in the usual community services condition (28%).[23] In another RCT evaluating (1) MST, (2) MST + contingency management (CM), (3) family court usual services, and (4) drug court usual services, cannabis use significantly decreased from pretreatment to 4 month and this decrease persisted at 12 months across treatments, with juvenile offenders in the 2 MST conditions reporting less cannabis use (3.7 and 6.8 days over the past 90 days) than those in the family court usual services condition (13.4 days).[24] In addition, juvenile offenders in the MST (28%) and MST + CM (18%) conditions had a significantly lower percent of positive cannabis drug screens than in the drug court usual services (69%) between pretreatment to 4 months and 4 months to 12 months (MST: 7%, MST + CM: 17%, usual services: 45%). Overall, adolescents receiving MST with and without CM reported less cannabis use and had greater rates of cannabis abstinence than the usual community services conditions.

Functional family therapy

Functional family therapy (FFT) concentrates on reducing substance use by identifying and modifying maladaptive family patterns related to adolescent substance use and integrating cognitive behavioral techniques.[25] Only 1 RCT on FFT examining cannabis-specific outcomes was identified. Findings from this RCT, which compared individual CBT, FFT, combined individual CBT + FFT, and a psychoeducational group intervention, revealed a significant decline in days using cannabis over time for the FFT (55% to 25% of days over the past 90 days) and combined conditions at 4-month follow-up (57% to 38%).[26] This reduction was maintained at the 7-month follow-up for the combined condition (36% of days) but not in the FFT condition (40%). A significant change from heavy to minimal use (ie, reported use <10% of days) was also observed in the FFT and combined group from pretreatment to 4-month follow-up and from pretreatment to 7-month follow-up.

Individual-Focused Psychotherapies

Several individual-focused psychotherapies (vs family/environment focused) have been studied, including cognitive behavioral therapy (CBT), motivational enhancement therapy (MET), and CM. These models—specifically individual and group-delivered CBT and MET/CBT—were deemed well-established treatments for adolescent SUDs in a prior review, with multicomponent packages involving CM (eg, MET/

CBT + CM) identified as probably efficacious pending further investigation.[8] RCTs examining individual-focused psychotherapies for adolescents with cannabis use are described in later discussion.

Individual cognitive behavioral therapy
CBT is a structured approach that includes exploring an adolescents' substance use patterns and applying skills (eg, cognitive restructuring, refusal skills, negative mood regulation) to reduce substance use.[27] Three RCTs[11,16,28] found that adolescents receiving individual CBT demonstrated significant reductions in cannabis use at post-treatment, 6-month, and 12-month follow-ups, and 26% of adolescents in 1 study had negative urine drug screens (UDS) for cannabis at follow-up.[16] However, in another RCT, adolescents receiving CBT did not show a significant decrease in number of days using cannabis over time.[26] Although a significant change from heavy to minimal use (ie, reported use <10% of days) from pretreatment to 4 months was found for the individual CBT condition, this change was not maintained at 7-month follow-up but was maintained for the FFT and FFT + CBT conditions. Across all 4 RCTs reviewed, CBT was found to be similarly efficacious to the comparison treatments, which were often other evidence-based treatments (eg, MDFT, FFT).

Motivational enhancement therapy/cognitive behavioral therapy
MET/CBT combines CBT and MET, which applies motivational interviewing skills to resolve adolescents' ambivalence and increase their motivation to reduce substance use while also conducting a functional analysis of their substance use behavior.[29,30] Several RCTs have examined MET/CBT using varying numbers of sessions and formats (ie, group, individual). MET/CBT5 (2 individual MET sessions plus 3 group CBT sessions) has demonstrated an increase in days of abstinence from cannabis and other substance use over 12 months, resulted in 23% to 27% of adolescents in "recovery" (ie, no past month substance use and living in the community) at 12 months in 2 trials, and performed similarly to other treatments (MDFT, MET/CBT12, MET/CBT12 + family components, adolescent community reinforcement approach [A-CRA]).[12] One RCT found that 44% of adolescents receiving MET/CBT7 (ie, MET/CBT5 plus 2 family sessions) were in "recovery" from all substances at 12 months.[31] MET/CBT12 extends MET/CBT5 with 7 additional group CBT sessions. In 2 RCTs,[12,32] MET/CBT12 demonstrated a significant reduction in cannabis use frequency during treatment and showed increased abstinence days over 12 months, with 17% of adolescents in "recovery" at 12 months in 1 study.[12]

Adolescent community reinforcement approach
A-CRA focuses on increasing an adolescent's engagement in the community through engaging with family, peers, school, work, and extracurricular activities that are incompatible with substance use and support recovery.[12,33] In 1 RCT, A-CRA showed an increase in abstinence days over 12 months and 34% of adolescents who received A-CRA were in "recovery" (ie, no past month cannabis or other substance use problems and living in the community) at 12 months.[12] In 2 RCTs comparing the effectiveness of assertive continuing care (ie, A-CRA plus case management) to usual continuing care, both studies found that adolescents in the assertive continuing care group were more likely to be abstinent from cannabis (52% vs 31% at 3 months; 41% vs 26% at 9 months).[33,34]

Contingency management
CM has been studied in several RCTs, often as an adjunct to other treatments. CM implementation varies, including on level of caregiver involvements. Two RCTs

examined a point-and-level system version of CM, whereby youth could select rewards from a menu in response to negative urine screens; rewards included both natural incentives provided by the caregiver (eg, access to cell phone) and therapist-delivered payments to purchase prizes (up to $100–$150 per youth). Adolescents in the CM condition demonstrated a significant decrease in positive UDS at follow-up assessment,[35,36] although this finding did not persist at 12-month follow-up in 1 RCT.[36] In a comparison of this CM component with family engagement strategies with usual drug court substance abuse treatment services, adolescents in the CM condition demonstrated a larger decrease in cannabis use, with the odds of a positive cannabis drug screen result increasing 94% for usual treatment and decreasing 18% for CM when comparing months 7 to 9 with months 1 to 3.[35]

In a voucher-based CM model, adolescents can earn incentives for negative UDS using an escalating schedule with vouchers increasing in amount with each consecutive negative drug screen. In 1 study, MST enhanced with voucher-based CM yielded reductions in cannabis use from pretreatment to 4- and 12-month follow-ups, with MST and MST + CM having a significantly lower percent of positive UDS between pretreatment to 4 months (18% MST + CM, 28% MST) and 4 months to 12 months (17% MST + CM, 7% MST) compared with usual community services (69% and 45%).[24] Two RCTs evaluated a clinic-delivered abstinence-based CM component that also entailed a caregiver-delivered home-based CM component, which involved developing a substance monitoring contract (SMC) wherein positive and negative consequences were implemented for substance abstinence and use.[32,37] In both studies, MET/CBT + abstinence-based CM/SMC showed greater continuous cannabis abstinence during treatment than the other treatments (eg, MET/CBT, MET/CBT + attendance-based CM). Adolescents in an MET/CBT + abstinence-based CM/SMC + family management group had greater mean weeks of cannabis abstinence (7.6 vs 5.1) and were more likely to achieve 8 or more weeks (53% vs 30%) and 10 or more weeks of continuous abstinence (50% vs 18%) compared with adolescents in an MET/CBT + attendance-based CM treatment.[37] MET/CBT + CM/SMC with or without a parent training curriculum had a larger proportion of adolescents achieve 2+ and 4+ weeks of abstinence compared with MET/CBT without CM.[32] Importantly, both studies also found that improvements observed during treatment did not persist at follow-up.

In the Fishbowl CM method[38] youth earn prize draws per an escalating schedule based on evidence of target behaviors (eg, negative UDS). Although no differences in cannabis abstinence rates were observed between treatments in an RCT evaluating (1) MET/CBT + abstinence-based CM/SMC + weekly behavioral parent training and (2) MET/CBT + attendance-based incentives, the abstinence-based condition had a significantly lower mean percentage of cannabis use days than the attendance-based condition at 36-week follow-up (27% vs 37%).[39] Another RCT compared CM + standard community treatment with a control group (ie, standard community treatment plus 2 prize draws for each drug screen submission independent of result) and did not find significant differences between groups in percent of negative UDS submitted (57% vs 42%) and sustained negative UDS (5.3 vs 5.1).[40]

Overall, CM seems to enhance cannabis use treatment outcomes, particularly when added to an evidence-based intervention and tied to cannabis use, but several studies show limited maintenance of effects once incentives are discontinued.[32,36,37]

Integrated Psychotherapies

Adolescents with SUDs frequently experience co-occurring psychiatric disorders.[41,42] Emerging evidence supports the safety and efficacy of integrated treatments designed to address both substance use and psychiatric disorders. Notably, several of the family-based therapies reviewed earlier have shown effects on externalizing problems in addition to cannabis and other substance use.[13,14,16,20]

Risk Reduction through Family Therapy (RRFT) is an integrative, ecologically informed, exposure-based treatment that addresses co-occurring trauma-related symptoms and risk behaviors, including substance use.[43] In an RCT comparing RRFT with treatment as usual (TAU) in adolescents with substance use and posttraumatic stress disorder (PTSD) symptoms, both conditions showed improved PTSD symptoms.[44] The RRFT group showed greater reductions than TAU in any cannabis use from baseline to 6 (−54% vs −21%), 12 (−71% vs −34%), and 18 months (−67% vs −1%). For number of cannabis use days, greater reductions were observed in the RRFT group from baseline (−4.4 days at 12 months and 18 months) compared with the TAU group (−0.7 days at 12 months, +2.1 days at 18 months).

Esposito-Smythers and colleagues (2011)[45] examined a family-based integrated CBT intervention (I-CBT) for adolescents with co-occurring SUD and suicidality compared with enhanced treatment-as-usual. The I-CBT condition showed a greater reduction in cannabis use days, less cannabis problems over time, and lower rates of overall SUDs (27% vs 77%) at the 18-month follow-up than the comparison group. Another RCT explored the effectiveness of home-based I-CBT relative to enhanced treatment-as-usual on substance use and psychiatric symptoms, but study findings were limited due to low power to detect effects.[46]

PHARMACOTHERAPIES FOR CANNABIS USE DISORDER IN ADOLESCENTS

To date, no medication has approval from the Food and Drug Administration for the treatment of CUD. Two drugs have been investigated in adolescents: N-acetylcysteine (NAC) and topiramate. NAC is an antioxidant derived from L-cysteine that may help youth quit using cannabis when combined with other therapeutic interventions. Gray and colleagues[47] conducted an open-label trial demonstrating NAC 1200 mg twice a day was safe and tolerable among youth (aged 18–21 years) with CUD. A subsequent RCT of NAC (1200 mg twice daily) combined with CM and brief weekly cessation counseling was conducted in treatment-seeking youth (aged 15–21 years) with cannabis dependence.[48] Among youth who received NAC, 40.9% of urine cannabinoid test results over the treatment period were negative compared with 27.7% of the placebo group (odds ratio [OR], 2.4; 95% confidence interval [CI], 1.1–5.2), with an estimated number needed to treat of 7.3. By 4-week posttreatment follow-up, negative urine tests decreased to 19.0% for the NAC group and 10.3% for the placebo group (OR, 2.4; 95% CI, 0.8–7.5). End of treatment abstinence favored NAC, although differences were not statistically significant (OR, 2.3; 95% CI, 1.0–5.4). A second RCT of NAC in treatment-seeking adults with CUD found no difference in negative UDS between treatment groups.[49] NAC is available as tablets or capsules and an oral solution. Anecdotally, in settings in which pill forms are not available (ie, inpatient hospitalization), most adolescents are not compliant with the liquid form due to taste intolerability.

Topiramate is a carbonic anhydrase inhibitor that results in potentiation of γ-aminobutyric acid (GABA) signaling and inhibition of glutamate and voltage-gated sodium and calcium channels.[50] Although primarily used for seizure disorders, migraines, and other chronic pain, clinical trials of topiramate have demonstrated reductions in alcohol, cocaine, and nicotine use in adults.[51–55] Miranda and colleagues[56] conducted a randomized placebo-controlled pilot study of topiramate combined with MET in individuals (aged 15–24 years) who were treatment-seeking heavy cannabis users (cannabis use at least twice weekly and 1 or more symptoms of CUD). Topiramate was titrated over 4 weeks and continued at 200 mg daily for 2 weeks. Although youth in the topiramate group reported greater reductions in grams of cannabis smoked per day, there were no differences in abstinence rates. Furthermore, only 48% of the topiramate group completed the study, compared with 77% of the placebo group, with adverse drug events being the most common reason for discontinuation. Secondary analysis found that memory difficulties were a predominant predictor of dropout in the topiramate group, in addition to other common cognitive side effects of topiramate (slow thinking, word finding difficulties, confusion).[57] Interestingly, youth with greater cannabis problems were less likely to drop out of the topiramate group. These findings suggest further investigation may be warranted for the targeted use of topiramate in heavy cannabis-using youth who are also experiencing impairing cannabis-related problems, although the side effect burden may limit topiramate's utility.

Numerous other drugs have been investigated for the treatment of CUD and/or cannabis withdrawal in adults.[6,7] First, 2 medications have been associated with a reduction in cannabis use: quetiapine and nabilone, a Schedule II synthetic tetrahydrocannabinol (THC) derivative. A recent RCT of quetiapine 300 mg daily versus placebo found quetiapine was associated with transition of heavy cannabis use (5–7 d/wk) to moderate use (2–4 d/wk).[58] However, at a dose of 200 mg/d, quetiapine was previously shown to increase cannabis craving and self-administration during relapse.[59] Second, cannabinoid agents may attenuate cannabis craving and withdrawal. Nabilone 8 mg/d was associated with reductions in amount of cannabis used and attenuation of cannabis withdrawal.[60] Other cannabinoid agents, including dronabinol (40–80 mg/d),[6,61] a THC derivative, and nabiximols,[62] a *Cannabis sativa* extract that contains both THC and CBD, have been shown to attenuate cannabis craving and withdrawal, respectively. Third, mirtazapine, a noradrenergic antidepressant, was shown to improve sleep, a common reason that individuals relapse to cannabis use, and food intake during abstinence in a human laboratory trial (30 mg/d).[63] Finally, multiple medications including noradrenergic agents atomoxetine, bupropion, and venlafaxine and GABAergic agents depakote and baclofen were poorly tolerated, resulting in high study attrition.[6,7] None of these agents have yet been studied in adolescent samples.

DISCUSSION

There are several evidence-supported treatment options available for youth with CUDs. These programs vary in their focus, intensity, and availability in the community, but they share an emphasis on addressing common maintaining factors for cannabis use. Many of the trials reviewed here were conducted before dramatic changes in the national landscape around cannabis use (eg, state-level legalization, proliferation of more potent cannabis products). THC concentrations in herbal cannabis and cannabis resin have increased steadily over the last 5 decades,[64] and many of the solutions, waxes, and concentrates used in e-cigarettes contain much higher THC concentrations (up to 80%) than dried cannabis leaves.[65] The use of vaporizers has made it easier for youth to use cannabis discretely in public spaces including schools.[66] Moreover, cannabis is increasingly viewed as safe and acceptable among adolescents.[67] Higher THC concentrations, coupled with greater ease of use and more permissive attitudes about cannabis use, may contribute to increased cannabis dependence and greater need for accessible, effective treatments.[68] Established interventions should continue to be tested for their efficacy to determine what adaptations may be needed in the current context. Interventions also should address key barriers to care, such as behavioral health workforce shortages.[69] New digital platforms that deliver evidence-based treatment components (eg, CBT, CM, behavior monitoring) to youth may be especially helpful if shown to facilitate treatment progress while also reducing clinician burden.[70] Given the potential for technology to improve the accessibility and effectiveness of interventions, more research in adolescent samples is sorely needed.

There is need for additional research into treatments designed specifically to address cannabis use, because few studies focused specifically on reducing cannabis use or CUD remission.[12,15,16,32,37,40] Although many risk and protective factors contribute to substance use broadly, directly addressing mechanisms uniquely associated with CUD may yield better effects. In addition, although existing treatments often produce improvements during treatment, there was frequently poor sustainment of effects, and not all adolescents responded to treatment. There is a lack of long-term follow-ups across studies, with most follow-up assessments concluding at or before 1 year. Considered together, these findings signal a need for further research into tailored interventions designed specifically to yield clinically meaningful, durable reductions in cannabis use in adolescents.

Clinical leaders and researchers should also consider implementation factors that may impact outcomes when selecting and testing CUD treatments. These considerations include costs and cost-effectiveness of delivering the treatment, the time and resources needed to achieve high treatment fidelity (eg, workshops, ongoing supervision or consultation, treatment manual), organizational barriers (eg, organizational culture, leadership), and external policies and regulations.[71] For example, Henggeler and colleagues (1999)[22] cited low treatment fidelity as a potential reason for smaller MST effects in 1 study. Such findings underscore the importance of addressing provider-, agency-, and system-level factors that can influence treatment outcomes so that interventions can achieve optimal effects. Where cost-effectiveness was examined in the RCTs reviewed here, MET/CBT was found to be the most cost-effective intervention option, which may increase the likelihood that the model will be adopted broadly.[12,31] Nearly all reviewed studies were conducted in outpatient settings, but youth with CUD may benefit from participating in treatments in other contexts like schools, primary care, and juvenile justice. The unique implementation challenges of each setting should be addressed either through adaptations to existing treatment models or through development of new interventions designed specifically for "nontraditional" settings.

Few pharmacotherapies have been tested for the treatment of CUD in adolescents, and fewer still have demonstrated efficacy. Although data on NAC are encouraging, more research is needed to determine for whom and under what conditions these therapies are likely to be most helpful in addressing CUD symptoms in youth. Several studies in adults showed negative effects of medications for cannabis use. Although it is common for research on pediatric psychopharmacology to lag behind adult studies (due to safety concerns, and so on), it is notable that for NAC, treatment effects were observed in adolescents but not in adults. It may be appropriate in some cases to develop and study medications specifically meant for youth with CUD even when positive effects on cannabis use or CUD symptoms are not observed in adults. If found to be safe and effective, such medications could have enormous impact on population health and well-being by curtailing the harms and costs associated with addiction early in development.

CLINICS CARE POINTS

- Manualized psychotherapies, including MET/CBT and various family-based treatments, target internal and external maintaining factors of cannabis use and can be effective in addressing CUD symptoms in adolescents when delivered with fidelity.

- Many treatments directly address youth ambivalence and/or directly reinforce engagement in treatment activities, so patients do not need to be committed to reducing or abstaining from cannabis use to be referred to treatment.
- Pharmacotherapies should be considered alongside psychotherapies to help youth with CUD manage cravings.

DISCLOSURE

The authors have nothing to disclose.

ACKNOWLEDGEMENT

The authors wish to acknowledge support from NIH grant K12DA000357 (JH) and SAMHSA grant H79TI083595 (ZWA, LAH).

REFERENCES

1. MTF MtF. 1975-2021 data for in-school Surveys of 8th, 10th, and 12th Grade students. University of Michigan. 2021. http://monitoringthefuture.org/data/21data.htm. [Accessed 15 January 2022].
2. Quality CfBHSa. National survey on drug Use and health, 2019 and Quarters 1 and 4, 2020. SAMHSA. https://www.samhsa.gov/data/sites/default/files/reports/rpt35323/NSDUHDetailedTabs2020/NSDUHDetailedTabs2020/NSDUHDetTabsSect5pe2020.htm. [Accessed 15 January 2022].
3. Silins E, Horwood LJ, Patton GC, et al. Young adult sequelae of adolescent cannabis use: an integrative analysis. The Lancet Psychiatry 2014;1(4):286–93.
4. Kosty DB, Seeley JR, Farmer RF, et al. Trajectories of cannabis use disorder: risk factors, clinical characteristics and outcomes. Addiction 2017;112(2):279–87.
5. Oshri A, Rogosch FA, Burnette ML, et al. Developmental pathways to adolescent cannabis abuse and dependence: Child maltreatment, emerging personality, and internalizing versus externalizing psychopathology. Psychol Addict Behaviors 2011;25(4):634–44.
6. Brezing CA, Levin FR. The current state of Pharmacological treatments for cannabis Use disorder and withdrawal. Neuropsychopharmacology 2018;43(1):173–94.
7. Kondo KK, Morasco BJ, Nugent SM, et al. Pharmacotherapy for the treatment of cannabis Use disorder. Ann Intern Med 2020;172(6):398–412.
8. Hogue A, Henderson CE, Becker SJ, et al. Evidence Base on outpatient behavioral treatments for adolescent substance Use, 2014–2017: outcomes, treatment delivery, and promising Horizons. J Clin Child Adolesc Psychol 2018;47(4):499–526.
9. Tanner-Smith EE, Wilson SJ, Lipsey MW. The comparative effectiveness of outpatient treatment for adolescent substance abuse: a meta-analysis. J Substance Abuse Treat 2013;44(2):145–58.
10. Liddle HA, Rodriguez RA, Dakof GA, et al. Multidimensional family therapy: a science-based treatment for adolescent drug abuse. Handbook Clin Fam Ther 2005;128–63.
11. Liddle HA, Dakof GA, Turner RM, et al. Treating adolescent drug abuse: a randomized trial comparing multidimensional family therapy and cognitive behavior therapy. Addiction 2008;103(10):1660–70.

12. Dennis M, Godley SH, Diamond G, et al. The Cannabis Youth Treatment (CYT) Study: main findings from two randomized trials. J Subst Abuse Treat 2004; 27(3):197–213.

13. Liddle HA, Dakof GA, Parker K, et al. Multidimensional family therapy for adolescent drug abuse: results of a randomized clinical trial. Am J Drug Alcohol Abuse 2001;27(4):651–88.

14. Liddle HA, Rowe CL, Dakof GA, et al. Early intervention for adolescent substance abuse: pretreatment to posttreatment outcomes of a randomized clinical trial comparing multidimensional family therapy and peer group treatment. J Psychoactive Drugs 2004;36(1):49–63.

15. Rigter H, Henderson CE, Pelc I, et al. Multidimensional family therapy lowers the rate of cannabis dependence in adolescents: a randomised controlled trial in Western European outpatient settings. Drug Alcohol Depend 2013;130(1–3): 85–93.

16. Hendriks V, van der Schee E, Blanken P. Treatment of adolescents with a cannabis use disorder: main findings of a randomized controlled trial comparing multidimensional family therapy and cognitive behavioral therapy in The Netherlands. Drug Alcohol Depend 2011;119(1–2):64–71.

17. Szapocznik J, Kurtines WM. Breakthroughs in family therapy with drug abusing and problem youth. Breakthroughs in family therapy with drug abusing and problem youth. New York: Springer Publishing Company; 1989. xiii, 191.

18. Santisteban DA, Coatsworth JD, Perez-Vidal A, et al. Efficacy of brief strategic family therapy in modifying Hispanic adolescent behavior problems and substance use. J Fam Psychol 2003;17(1):121–33.

19. Robbins MS, Feaster DJ, Horigian VE, et al. Brief strategic family therapy versus treatment as usual: results of a multisite randomized trial for substance using adolescents. J Consult Clin Psychol 2011;79(6):713–27.

20. Horigian VE, Feaster DJ, Robbins MS, et al. A cross-sectional assessment of the long term effects of brief strategic family therapy for adolescent substance use. Am J Addict 2015;24(7):637–45.

21. Henggeler SW, Schoenwald SK, Borduin CM, et al. Multisystemic therapy for antisocial behavior in children and adolescents. New York: Guilford Press; 2009.

22. Henggeler SW, Pickrel SG, Brondino MJ. Multisystemic treatment of substance-abusing and-dependent delinquents: outcomes, treatment fidelity, and transportability. Ment Health Serv Res 1999;1(3):171–84.

23. Henggeler SW, Clingempeel WG, Brondino MJ, et al. Four-year follow-up of Multisystemic therapy with substance-abusing and substance-dependent juvenile offenders. J Am Acad Child Adolesc Psychiatry 2002;41(7):868–74.

24. Henggeler SW, Halliday-Boykins CA, Cunningham PB, et al. Juvenile drug court: enhancing outcomes by integrating evidence-based treatments. J Consult Clin Psychol 2006;74(1):42–54.

25. Alexander J, Parsons BV. Functional family therapy. Functional family therapy. Carmel, CA: Brooks/Cole Publishing Company; 1982. x, 188-x, 188.

26. Barrett H, Slesnick N, Brody JL, et al. Treatment outcomes for adolescent substance abuse at 4- and 7-month assessments. J Consulting Clin Psychol 2001; 69(5):802–13.

27. Beck AT, Wright FW, Newman CF, et al. Cognitive therapy of substance abuse. New York: Guilford Press; 1993.

28. Azrin NH, Donahue B, Teichner GA, et al. A controlled evaluation and Description of individual-cognitive problem Solving and family-behavior therapies in Dually-

Diagnosed Conduct-Disordered and substance-dependent youth. Article. J Child Adolesc Substance Abuse 2001;11(1):1.

29. Sampl S, Kadden R. Motivational enhancement therapy and cognitive behavioral therapy for adolescent cannabis users: 5 sessions, cannabis youth treatment (CYT) Series, vol. 1. Rockville, MD: Center for Substance Abuse Treatment, Substance Abuse and Mental Health Services Administration; 2001.

30. Webb C, Scudder M, Kaminer Y, et al. Motivational enhancement therapy and cognitive behavioral therapy Supplement: 7 sessions of cognitive behavioral therapy for adolescent cannabis users, cannabis youth treatment (CYT) Series, vol. 2. Center for Substance Abuse Treatment, Substance Abuse and Mental Health Services Administration; 2002.

31. Godley SH, Garner BR, Passetti LL, et al. Adolescent outpatient treatment and continuing care: main findings from a randomized clinical trial. Drug Alcohol Depend 2010;110(1–2):44–54.

32. Stanger C, Ryan SR, Scherer EA, et al. Clinic- and home-based contingency management plus parent training for adolescent cannabis use disorders. J Am Acad Child Adolesc Psychiatry 2015;54(6):445–453 e2.

33. Godley MD, Godley SH, Dennis ML, et al. The effect of assertive continuing care on continuing care linkage, adherence and abstinence following residential treatment for adolescents with substance use disorders. Addiction 2007;102(1): 81–93.

34. Godley MD, Godley SH, Dennis ML, et al. Preliminary outcomes from the assertive continuing care experiment for adolescents discharged from residential treatment. J Substance Abuse Treat 2002;23(1):21–32.

35. Henggeler SW, McCart MR, Cunningham PB, et al. Enhancing the effectiveness of juvenile drug courts by integrating evidence-based practices. J Consult Clin Psychol 2012;80(2):264–75.

36. Letourneau EJ, McCart MR, Sheidow AJ, et al. First evaluation of a contingency management intervention addressing adolescent substance Use and Sexual risk behaviors: risk reduction therapy for adolescents. J Subst Abuse Treat 2017;72: 56–65.

37. Stanger C, Budney AJ, Kamon JL, et al. A randomized trial of contingency management for adolescent marijuana abuse and dependence. Drug Alcohol Depend 2009;105(3):240–7.

38. Petry NM. A comprehensive guide to the application of contingency management procedures in clinical settings. Drug and Alcohol Dependence 2000;58(1):9–25.

39. Stanger C, Scherer EA, Babbin SF, et al. Abstinence based incentives plus parent training for adolescent alcohol and other substance misuse. Psychol Addict Behav 2017;31(4):385–92.

40. Killeen TK, McRae-Clark AL, Waldrop AE, et al. Contingency management in community programs treating adolescent substance abuse: a feasibility study. J Child Adolesc Psychiatr Nurs 2012;25(1):33–41.

41. Armstrong TD, Costello EJ. Community studies on adolescent substance use, abuse, or dependence and psychiatric comorbidity. J Consulting Clin Psychol 2002;70(6):1224–39.

42. Chan Y-F, Dennis ML, Funk RR. Prevalence and comorbidity of major internalizing and externalizing problems among adolescents and adults presenting to substance abuse treatment. J Substance Abuse Treat 2008;34(1):14–24.

43. Danielson CK, Adams ZA, Hanson R. Risk reduction through family therapy (RRFT): exposure-based treatment for co-occurring PTSD and substance use problems among adolescents. In: Vujanovic AA, Back SE, editors. Posttraumtic

stress and substance Use disorders: a Comprehensive clinical Handbook. Routledge; 2019. p. 165–82.

44. Danielson CK, Adams Z, McCart MR, et al. Safety and efficacy of exposure-based risk reduction through family therapy for Co-occurring substance Use problems and Posttraumatic stress disorder symptoms among adolescents: a randomized clinical trial. JAMA Psychiatry 2020;77(6):574–86.

45. Esposito-Smythers C, Spirito A, Kahler CW, et al. Treatment of co-occurring substance abuse and suicidality among adolescents: a randomized trial. J Consult Clin Psychol 2011;79(6):728–39.

46. Wolff J, Esposito-Smythers C, Frazier E, et al. A randomized trial of an integrated cognitive behavioral treatment protocol for adolescents receiving home-based services for co-occurring disorders. J Subst Abuse Treat 2020;116:108055.

47. Gray KM, Watson NL, Carpenter MJ, et al. N-acetylcysteine (NAC) in young marijuana users: an open-label pilot study. Am J Addict 2010;19(2):187–9.

48. Gray KM, Carpenter MJ, Baker NL, et al. A double-blind randomized controlled trial of N-acetylcysteine in cannabis-dependent adolescents. Am J Psychiatry 2012;169(8):805–12.

49. Gray KM, Sonne SC, McClure EA, et al. A randomized placebo-controlled trial of N-acetylcysteine for cannabis use disorder in adults. Drug and Alcohol Dependence 2017;177:249–57.

50. Shank RP, Gardocki JF, Streeter AJ, et al. An overview of the preclinical aspects of topiramate: pharmacology, pharmacokinetics, and mechanism of action. Epilepsia 2000;41(S1):3–9.

51. Johnson BA, Ait-Daoud N, Bowden CL, et al. Oral topiramate for treatment of alcohol dependence: a randomised controlled trial. Lancet 2003;361(9370):1677–85.

52. Miranda R Jr, MacKillop J, Monti PM, et al. Effects of topiramate on urge to drink and the subjective effects of alcohol: a preliminary laboratory study. Alcohol Clin Exp Res 2008;32(3):489–97.

53. Johnson BA, Ait-Daoud N, Wang XQ, et al. Topiramate for the treatment of cocaine addiction: a randomized clinical trial. JAMA psychiatry 2013;70(12):1338–46.

54. Kranzler HR, Covault J, Feinn R, et al. Topiramate treatment for heavy drinkers: moderation by a GRIK1 polymorphism. Am J Psychiatry 2014;171(4):445–52.

55. Oncken C, Arias AJ, Feinn R, et al. Topiramate for smoking cessation: a randomized, placebo-controlled pilot study. Nicotine Tob Res 2014;16(3):288–96.

56. Miranda R, Treloar H, Blanchard A, et al. Topiramate and motivational enhancement therapy for cannabis use among youth: a randomized placebo-controlled pilot study. Addict Biol 2017;22(3):779–90.

57. Gray JC, Treloar Padovano H, Wemm SE, et al. Predictors of topiramate Tolerability in heavy cannabis-using adolescents and young adults: a secondary analysis of a randomized, double-blind, placebo-controlled trial. J Clin Psychopharmacol 2018;38(2):134–7.

58. Mariani JJ, Pavlicova M, Jean Choi C, et al. Quetiapine treatment for cannabis use disorder. Drug and Alcohol Dependence 2021;218:108366.

59. Cooper ZD, Foltin RW, Hart CL, et al. A human laboratory study investigating the effects of quetiapine on marijuana withdrawal and relapse in daily marijuana smokers. Addict Biol 2013;18(6):993–1002.

60. Haney M, Cooper ZD, Bedi G, et al. Nabilone decreases marijuana withdrawal and a laboratory measure of marijuana relapse. Neuropsychopharmacology 2013;38(8):1557–65.

61. Levin FR, Mariani JJ, Brooks DJ, et al. Dronabinol for the treatment of cannabis dependence: a randomized, double-blind, placebo-controlled trial. Drug and Alcohol Dependence 2011;116(1–3):142–50.
62. Allsop DJ, Copeland J, Lintzeris N, et al. Nabiximols as an agonist replacement therapy during cannabis withdrawal: a randomized clinical trial. JAMA psychiatry 2014;71(3):281–91.
63. Haney M, Hart CL, Vosburg SK, et al. Effects of baclofen and mirtazapine on a laboratory model of marijuana withdrawal and relapse. Psychopharmacology (Berl) 2010;211(2):233–44.
64. Freeman TP, Craft S, Wilson J, et al. Changes in delta-9-tetrahydrocannabinol (THC) and cannabidiol (CBD) concentrations in cannabis over time: systematic review and meta-analysis. Addiction 2021;116(5):1000–10. https://doi.org/10.1111/add.15253.
65. Meier MH, Docherty M, Leischow SJ, et al. Cannabis concentrate Use in adolescents. Pediatrics 2019;144(3):e20190338.
66. Ramamurthi D, Chau C, Jackler RK. JUUL and other stealth vaporisers: hiding the habit from parents and teachers. Tob Control 2019;28(6):610.
67. Schulenberg JE, Patrick ME, Johnston LD, et al. Monitoring the Future national survey results on drug use, 1975–2020: Volume II, College students and adults ages 19–60. 2021. http://www.monitoringthefuture.org/pubs/monographs/mtf-vol2_2020.pdf. [Accessed 15 January 2022].
68. Freeman TP, Winstock AR. Examining the profile of high-potency cannabis and its association with severity of cannabis dependence. Psychol Med 2015;45(15):3181–9.
69. U.S. Department of Health and Human Services HRaSA, National Center for Health Workforce Analysis. State-level Projections of supply and Demand for behavioral health Occupations: 2016-2030 2018.
70. Hammond AS, Sweeney MM, Chikosi TU, et al. Digital delivery of a contingency management intervention for substance use disorder: a feasibility study with DynamiCare Health. J Substance Abuse Treat 2021;126:108425. https://doi.org/10.1016/j.jsat.2021.108425.
71. Damschroder LJ, Aron DC, Keith RE, et al. Fostering implementation of health services research findings into practice: a consolidated framework for advancing implementation science. Implementation Sci 2009;4(1):50.

National Institute on Drug Abuse

Dissemination of Scientific Knowledge to Improve Adolescent Health

Geetha A. Subramaniam, MD[a],*, Laura Nolan, BA[b],
Kristen Huntley, PhD[a], Michelle Corbin, MBA[a],
Kenyatta Crenshaw, MEd[c], Todd Mandell, MD[c],
Janet Linton, MSM[a,d], Quandra Blackeney, BS[a]

KEYWORDS

- Dissemination • Adolescent health • Substance use • Provider education
- Addiction

KEY POINTS

- Timely and wide translation of NIDA's science and research findings is necessary to educate health care providers (HCPs), and to inform policy makers and youth and their families, and it ultimately improves adolescent and public health.
- NIDA's web portals such as NIDAMED, CTN Dissemination Initiative, Research Studies/ Translational Research Resources (Drug Topics), NIDA for Teens, and CTN Dissemination Library disseminate empirically based evidence regarding adolescent substance use.
- Dissemination of scientific information involves active partnerships with researchers; professional organizations; youth and their families; and educators and policy makers, to ensure bidirectional exchange, and to inform a constantly evolving process to make relevant information readily available in user-friendly and cost-free formats.

This article originally appeared in *Child and Adolescent Psychiatric Clinics*, Volume 32 Issue 1, January 2023.
[a] Center for the Clinical Trials Network, National Institute on Drug Abuse, 3WFN RM 09A54 MSC 6022, 301 North Stonestreet Avenue, Bethesda, MD 20892, USA; [b] JBS International, Inc., 5515 Security Lane, North Bethesda, MD 20852, USA; [c] The Bizzell Group LLC, 8201 Corporate Drive, 9th Floor, New Carrollton, MD 20785, USA; [d] Center for Tobacco Products, U.S. Food and Drug Administration, 10903 New Hampshire Avenue, Silver Spring, MD 20993, USA
* Corresponding author. 11601 Landsdown Street, MSC 6022 Bethesda, Maryland 20892, USA
E-mail address: geetha.subramaniam@nih.gov

INTRODUCTION/BACKGROUND

The National Institute on Drug Abuse's (NIDA) mission is to advance the science on the causes and consequences of drug use and addiction and to apply that knowledge to improve individual and public health. Crucial to this mission is the wide and effective translation and dissemination of research findings achieved via a variety of approaches tailored for target audiences, which will be the focus of this article.

It is widely reported that it takes approximately 17 years for research evidence to make its way to day-to-day clinical practice, depriving adults and youth of timely and appropriate clinical care.[1] There are several barriers to dissemination at the patient level (eg, lack of patient involvement in the proposed research, use of narrow eligibility criteria in clinical trials), provider level (limited access to publications in research journals, limited educational and training opportunities for clinical staff, reluctance to treat youth with substance use problems, stigma); and organizational/system level (eg, stigma, lack of resources, inadequate reimbursement, lack of the prioritization of substance use needs, and so forth). In 2016, NIH published a policy (https://bit.ly/NOT-OD-16-149) on the dissemination of NIH-funded clinical research requiring that all clinical trial investigators register and submit summary results to ClincalTrials.gov for public posting, as a means to advance the translation of research findings.[2] However, successful communication of scientific knowledge to the community requires additional efforts. Given the vast scope of materials and approaches to NIDA dissemination efforts, in this article, we focus on initiatives/campaigns and web portals pertaining to adolescent substance use. These resources are divided into 3 categories: I. clinician/health care provider (HCP) education; II. research studies and translational research resources (drug topics); and III. materials for teens, families, and educators. The resources described in this article, and other content on the NIDAMED website, are available at no cost and may be freely reproduced for educational/research purposes. We also notify the readers that NIDA websites are regularly assessed for relevance and utility, resulting in a dynamic process whereby new content is created, and existing content is either updated or removed (so website links at the time of this publication may not be functional in the future).

APPROACH
Educational Resources for Clinicians/Health Care Providers

In addition to conducting and funding cutting-edge basic and clinical research on addiction, NIDA aims to transfer this scientific knowledge into clinical practice and disseminate it broadly. A substantial portion of NIDA's mission to disseminate science is executed through NIDAMED, an initiative that connects adolescent health professionals and other HCPs with science-based information, resources, tools, and training on substance use disorder (SUD), screening, prevention, intervention, and treatment that can be applied in the direct care of their patients. The NIDAMED website (drugabuse.gov/nidamed) is a portal for HCPs and those in training to access science-based resources on addressing addiction in practice. Through various methods, including communication with panels of HCPs, partnerships with key health care professional organizations, online surveys, and semi-structured interviews, the NIDAMED initiative seeks to identify HCPs' needs for information about addiction and their communication preferences for receiving this information. This feedback loop allows NIDAMED to develop targeted resources and dissemination strategies that increase awareness of the resources, information, and products available for HCPs on addiction.

Fostering partnerships with medical professional organizations that represent HCPs is key to the success of the NIDAMED initiative. Through these partnerships, NIDA is able to develop and share with partners and their members the most up-to-date, evidence-based resources on addiction. Partnerships and information sharing with these organizations have taken many forms, from holding webinars with their members with NIDA staff, to writing articles for their magazines, to partnering on awareness events (eg, American Society of Addiction Medicine's [ASAM] Addiction Treatment Week), to participating/speaking at meetings and conferences, to interviewing members for spotlight pieces, to working together on systematic reviews, and more.

Dissemination of NIDAMED's resources is conducted via multiple channels, including monthly and ad hoc e-blasts to 87,000+ HCPs; NIDA's social media platforms (eg, Twitter, LinkedIn); and communications (eg, social media posts, newsletters, magazines, webinars) from partners (eg, medical professional organizations) to their members. Through these dissemination efforts, past year sessions on the NIDAMED web portal increased by 26.03% to 399,828 when compared with the 317,259 sessions recorded from the previous year. Resources outlined in this section were generally disseminated via these channels unless otherwise noted.

Key components of the NIDAMED web portal are highlighted below to include (a) NIDA-funded SUD screening tools; (b) Medical Health Professionals Education; (c) National Drug Abuse Treatment Clinical Trials Network's Dissemination Initiative; (d) CTN Dissemination Library; (e) Science to Medicine: Clinicians in Action; (f) Information on Stigma and Health Disparities; and (g) Resources on SUD Prevention and Treatment.

National Institute on Drug Abuse-funded substance use disorder screening tools

The American Academy of Pediatrics recommends universal screening in pediatric primary care settings, as it provides a unique opportunity to address substance use with their patients and families. To address this need, 2 NIDA-funded, brief, validated screening tools, Screening to Brief Intervention (S2BI)[3] and Brief Screener for Tobacco, Alcohol and other Drugs (BSTAD)[4] which providers can use to assess SUD risk among adolescents 12 to 17 years old, have been posted online. They are both briefs, empirically validated, and self- or-clinician administered electronically. Both the BSTAD and S2BI (https://bit.ly/BstadS2bi) ask patients about the frequency of past year use and triage them into one of the 3 levels of SUD risk: no reported use, lower risk, and higher risk. The implications of scores and suggested actions, based on subject matter expert consensus, are available to guide treatment planning.

Medical health professionals' education

NIDAMED also offers educational materials for preceptors and providers to expand their knowledge and stay up-to-date on the latest trends in substance use and addiction. Following are a few notes on adolescent SUD, several of which offer continuing medical education (CME) credit for providers:

- The Research-based Clinical Strategies to Prevent and Address Adolescent Substance Use and Prescription Medication Misuse: Being Part of the Solution course (https://bit.ly/TeenSUCME) aims to help providers navigate confidentiality in discussions with adolescent patients about their substance use; it includes provider videos and tips and talking points for patients at all risk levels. NIDAMED convened a coalition of HCPs and organizations (the Coalition) to inform the development of this course. More than 28,000 HCPs participated in the course, with more than 15,160 receiving a certificate of completion. This course was disseminated through the Coalition and partner organizations, NIDA's dissemination channels, and via Peer-Audience.com—an organization focusing on audience generation for CME activities.

- The Centers of Excellence for Physician Information website offers supplemental curriculum resources (CRs) for preceptors, with one focused on the adolescent population. The web-based module, Substance Use Disorders in Adolescents: Screening and Engagement in Primary Care Settings (https://bit.ly/NIDATeenCR) offers educational tools to assist in the prevention, screening, evaluation, and referral to the treatment of adolescents with or at risk for SUDs and includes a video and facilitator's guide. Results from a study on this module indicated that residents who were exposed to the CR had increased confidence in the efficacy of SUD treatment and their preparedness to care for patients with SUD. HCPs' attitudes and skills—enhanced from exposure to this CR—can help improve patient care.[5] CRs were disseminated via NIDAMED's channels, via medical schools who authored them, and through Mededportal.org.
- In collaboration with The Addiction Medicine Foundation, NIDAMED has created the Addiction Medicine Toolkit for Health Care Providers in Training. Designed as an introduction for health care providers (HCPs) in training before entering their fellowship programs, these resources can help prepare them for their journey to becoming certified in Addiction Medicine
- The Science to Medicine Series and Engaging Adolescent Patients About Marijuana (described later in discussion) are also accredited to offer CME credit.
- Publications; CMEs and other courses; and resources specific to Pediatricians on opioids, marijuana, treatment, and prevention are also compiled on the Discipline Spotlight: Pediatrician's page (https://bit.ly/DSPeds).

National drug abuse treatment clinical trials network's dissemination initiative

The CTN DI (https://bit.ly/CTNDI) aims to reduce the persistent gap between the publication of research findings on the treatment of SUDs and implementation, and adoption in clinical practice, of interventions and strategies grounded in that research evidence. (Although focused mainly on CTN studies, it also includes other NIDA research.) The initiative's resources are developed and disseminated through partnerships among researchers, clinicians, and trainers/stakeholders, in addition to inclusion on the NIDAMED website.

Following are examples of CTN DI resources on adolescent substance use:

- Engaging adolescent patients about Marijuana - This online interactive, avatar-based, learning module provides the user with an introduction to Motivational Interviewing (MI) within the pediatric primary care setting. It includes a brief overview of MI and an interactive role-play conversation with a virtual patient. Through this conversation, the user experiences how the spirit of MI can be used in appointments with adolescent patients who report marijuana use. Reported users of this resource include social workers, nurses, and medical and osteopathic doctors. For the year 2020, there were 5015 health care professionals who received CME/CE credit. In the first and second quarters of 2021 (January–June 2021), 1437 health care professionals obtained CME/CE credit.
- Mentor-Facilitated Training Awards (MFT) in Substance Use Disorders Science Dissemination (https://bit.ly/CTNDI) – This CTN DI initiative aims to enhance trainee HCP expertise in SUD dissemination activities. Trainees are funded for a year to conduct a project, through a mentoring experience, and disseminate the findings at their respective professional society annual meetings and publish them in a scientific journal. The awardees can also present their findings to their peers and within their local communities to help minimize gaps in current knowledge and practices. These awards are made available in partnership with participating health care professional organizations. Goals of the program include

teaching awardees more about SUD and supporting innovative ways to address gaps in current knowledge. The MFT program has partnered with several health care organizations since 2012, 2 of which target professionals working with adolescents such as the American Academy of Child and Adolescent Psychiatry, and the Society for Adolescent Health and Medicine. Additional health care organizations that have been in partnership with the MFT program include the: American College of Emergency Physicians/Emergency Medicine Foundation, Society of Teachers of Family Medicine, American Academy of Physician Assistants, American Association of Colleges of Nursing, American Association of Nurse Practitioners, and the Society of General Internal Medicine. Awardees have selected topics that focused on the treatment, screening, and prevention of SUDs involving (but not limited to) alcohol, tobacco, marijuana, and opioids. Many of the dissemination projects have resulted in the development of highly impactful training series, workshop curricula, and innovative technological tools/resources.

d) *CTN Dissemination Library* (https://bit.ly/CTNLibrary) – This CTN initiative consists of a digital repository of resources created by and about the CTN. It provides CTN members and the public with a single point of access to research findings and other materials. The Dissemination Library provides detailed information on CTN studies/protocols, dissemination products, the CTN Bulletin, presentations, workshops and webinars, and links to the CTN study pages and to the NIDA data share website. Examples of detailed information on completed CTN studies with youth are as follows:

o CTN 0028 osmotic-release methylphenidate for ADHD in adolescents with substance use disorders (https://bit.ly/CTN0028). The primary objective of this multisite, RCT was to evaluate the efficacy of OROS-MPH (Concerta), relative to placebo, in treating attention-deficit/hyperactivity disorder (ADHD) and decreasing substance use in adolescents with ADHD and a SUD.

o CTN-0010 - buprenorphine/naloxone-facilitated rehabilitation for opioid dependent adolescents/young adults (https://bit.ly/CTN-0010). The objective of this study was to compare buprenorphine/naloxone (Bup/Nx) treatment of 9 weeks and taper for 3 weeks to treatment as usual (Bup/Nx detox for 2 weeks). Both arms received counseling for 12 weeks.

o CTN-0014 - brief strategic family therapy (BSFT) for adolescent drug abusers (https://bit.ly/CTN-0014). This study was designed to compare BSFT to treatment as usual.

Science to medicine: clinicians in Action

Taking the latest research and sharing insights from clinicians about implementing it in clinical practice, Science to Medicine (STM) features real-world examples from a variety of practice settings and clinician types—operationalizing research to improve patient care. Working with partners at medical professional organizations, NIDAMED was able to identify and connect with pioneers in the field who were then interviewed by the NIDAMED team. These resources have been disseminated broadly and with the assistance of partnership organizations and the HCPs interviewees to their networks. Following are STM stories developed for adolescent HCPs.

• *Screening for Substance Use in the Pediatric/Adolescent Medicine Setting* (https://bit.ly/STMScreen). Adolescent Medicine providers Jennifer George Caffaro, PA-C, Physician Assistant, University of Kentucky HealthCare, Kentucky Children's Hospital, and Dawn Garzon Maaks, PhD, CPNP, PNP-BC, PMHS,

FAANP, Nurse Practitioner, LifeStance Health, St. Peters and Chesterfield, Missouri, discussed their screening practices; workflow for a typical patient; facilitators and barriers to screening and referral; and success stories. Their stories offer tips and considerations for other providers on screening adolescents for substance use—including how to get started and what to do with a positive screen.

- *Medication Treatment for Opioid Use Disorder (OUD) in the Pediatric (Adolescent Medicine) Setting* (https://bit.ly/STMTreat). Deepa Camenga, MD, Pediatrician and Addiction Medicine Specialist, Assistant Professor, Yale School of Medicine, describes her experiences with treating her adolescent patients with OUD, using Medications for OUD, in a primary care setting. She shared tips and considerations for other providers on how to get started.

Information on stigma and health disparities

People with SUDs face discrimination and negative bias from society, including from people who provide health care or other services in the community. Stereotypes that generate prejudice, and ultimately discrimination, stem from misinformed beliefs about addiction. Unfortunately, stigmatizing views of people with SUD are common; this stereotyping can lead others to feel pity, fear, anger, and a desire for social distance from people with a SUD. Stigmatizing language can negatively influence HCPs or professional perceptions of people with SUD, which can impact the care they provide.[6,7] Although some language that may be considered stigmatizing is commonly used within social communities of people who struggle with SUD, HCPs can show leadership in how language can destigmatize the disease of addiction. On the Addressing Stigma and Health Disparities page (bit.ly/StigmaPage), there are resources for HCPs including links to scientific publications, the NIDA director's blog on stigma, as well as quick facts, some of which were developed in partnership with other Federal agencies (eg, NIAAA). The seminal resource on this page, Words Matter: Terms to Use and Avoid When Talking about Addiction (https://bit.ly/WordsMatterHCP), was developed from identifying a need in conversation with partner organization, American Pharmacists Association. The language guide offers background information and tips for providers to keep in mind while using person-first language, terms to avoid to reduce stigma and negative bias when discussing addiction, and research-based reasons for using one term versus another. NIDAMED saw a need for (and developed) similar guides for (1) HCPs who treat pregnant women and mothers, featuring stories from women with SUD (https://bit.ly/WomensWordsMatter) and (2) the general public (https://bit.ly/WordsMatterPublic)—to learn more about what stigma is, how it affects people with SUD, and how to make a change. In 2020, the Association of American Medical Colleges held a webinar on MTV's documentary series *16 and Recovering*, which told the story of a Recovery high school and its students, and this Words Matter guide was linked to the documentary's webpage. These resources were widely distributed by partners and through NIDAMED channels—and continue to be extremely popular among HCPs.

Resources on substance use disorder prevention and treatment

Prevention efforts can help reduce adolescent substance use and the negative effects associated with substance use.[8] NIDAMED's Screening and Prevention page (https://bit.ly/NIDAPrevention) also provides links to prevention resources for providers to learn about evidence-based substance use prevention strategies—including a guide on substance use prevention in early childhood, adolescents, and young adults and a guide on how to dispose of unused medicine. Another NIDA publication, NIDA Notes "Preventive Interventions Delivered in Childhood May Reduce Substance Use Over

Two Generations" (bit.ly/ChildSUDPrevent) provides a distilled synopsis of The Raising Healthy Children (RHC) study, administered to children grades 1 to 6 at elementary schools in disadvantaged Seattle neighborhoods along with specialized training for teachers, parents, and children. Children of RHC recipients showed improved developmental functioning before age 5, as well as fewer problem behaviors; better academic, cognitive, and emotional skills; less risk behavior from ages 6 to 18; and sustained positive impact between ages 21 to 27, in the areas of education, employment, mental health, crime rates, and socio-economic attainment.

Treatment information is made available through infographics, links to resources, and publications of guides. An example of the latter is the Principles of Adolescent Substance Use Disorder Treatment: A Research-Based Guide (https://bit.ly/PrinciplesGuide). This is a comprehensive reference document that lists 13 principles of adolescent SUD treatment; provides a summary description of various SUD treatment settings; summarizes evidence-based behavioral, family-based, medication, and recovery support services; and links to treatment referral resources and answers to frequently asked questions.

Research and Translational Research Resources

In this section, we highlight 2 resources that clinicians may access to gain the most up-to-date information on: (1) 2 large longitudinal studies and (2) translational research resources (titled drug topics), which provide the most up-to-date information on drug use, trends, brain development, and outcomes. Regular updates on progress related to these studies and other relevant substance use research are shared via NIDA's social media and e-news communication channels.

a) *Monitoring the Future Study (MTF)* (https://bit.ly/MTFStudy) - Since 1975, this annual, NIDA-funded survey, conducted by researchers at the University of Michigan, Ann Arbor, has measured drug and alcohol use and related attitudes among eighth, 10th, and 12th grade students.[9] A nationally representative sample of survey participants report their drug use behaviors across 3 time periods: lifetime, past year, and past month.

More than 11,800 students from 112 schools across the United States participated in the 2020 survey. One example of the key 2020 MTF findings is that while there was a dramatic increase in the 30-day prevalence of any vaping (nicotine and/or marijuana) by adolescents, in the 2017 to 2019 surveys, rates had leveled and even reversed some in 2020. Trends in use among a nationwide sample of middle and high school students provide valuable information about opportunities for prevention/treatment, help measure the impact of prevention strategies, and may be used to shape future directions at NIDA, and by other key health care and policy stakeholders. NIDA also disseminates infographics (https://bit.ly/MTFInfographics), annually, after the results of the MTF survey are released, which serve as valuable visual aids for education and dissemination purposes.

b) *Adolescent Brain Cognitive Development*[SM] *Study (ABCD Study)* (https://bit.ly/ABCDNIDAStudy)- The ABCD study is the largest long-term study of brain development and child health ever conducted in the United States. The objectives of this ongoing study are to recruit 11,900 healthy children, ages 9 to 10 across the United States, with the goal of retaining 10,000 into early adulthood; use advanced brain imaging to observe brain growth with unprecedented precision; and examine how biology and environment interact and relate to developmental outcomes such as physical health, mental health, and life achievements including academic success. The results of this project will increase our understanding of environmental, social, genetic, substance use, and other biological factors (such as physical activity, screen time, and sleep, mental illness, state and local policies, and so forth) that affect the brain and cognitive development and that can impact children's/adolescents' life trajectories.

c) Drug topics: translational research resources

Each Drug Topics webpage includes a brief overview of a commonly used substance effect on the brain and body; statistics and trends; and relevant publications and articles written by NIDA researchers and scientists. Select Drug Topics resources on substances commonly used by youth are highlighted later in discussion:

- Marijuana (https://bit.ly/DrugTopicsMJ). This section offers a wealth of scientific facts regarding cannabis, including marijuana concentrates. Very briefly we list the content areas: describing what marijuana is, how it is used, types of marijuana extracts (eg, hash, wax, and so forth), short-term and long-term use of cannabis on the developing adolescent brain and physical health, as well as information on NIDA marijuana research; data on the rising potency and emerging variations of the marijuana products; and methods of use. Infographics on drugged driving and cannabis use trends featuring data from the MTF survey provide visual aids to convey the science to a broader audience.
- Tobacco/Nicotine Vaping (https://bit.ly/TobaccoNicconeVape). Here you will find drug facts on vaping devices (electronic cigarettes) and a publication on managing tobacco addiction. Also included is a Tobacco, Nicotine, and E-Cigarettes Research Report, a valuable guide covering a range of pertinent issues such as the impact of tobacco on youth and society, how tobacco delivers its effect, effects of secondhand and thirdhand smoke, and tobacco use trends. The NIDAMED web portal on Vaping, Marijuana, and Other Drugs (https://bit.ly/MJandVaping) is another resource on this topic. This portal was created to offer recent news and emerging trends related to vaping, based on recent trends (ie, last 5 years) from the MTF Study showing increased use of vaping and marijuana among adolescents.
- Alcohol (https://bit.ly/AlcoholDrugTopic). The Alcohol Drug Facts page provides links to information on alcohol and alcohol use disorder, treatment, research, and prevention. NIDA works closely with the National Institute on Alcohol Abuse and Alcoholism (NIAAA), the lead NIH institute supporting and conducting research on the impact of alcohol use on human health and well-being and the dissemination of these findings. NIDA funds research on the couse of alcohol with marijuana, opioids, and other substances and provides updates on the MTF survey results on alcohol use (https://bit.ly/AlcoholTrendsStats).

Resources and Information for Teens, Families, and Educators

Teens today confront many challenges in avoiding drug use. Rates of trauma and mental health disorders are high,[10] and teen suicide rates have increased in the past decade.[11] Legal cannabis, counterfeit pills, and vaping present new substance use opportunities for teens. Educating teens and their families about drug use and addiction is paramount to supporting prevention.

Educational resources from NIDA. NIDA Ed offers timely content on priority health topics, including multimedia educational resources, skills-based lessons, health-education standards-mapped prevention resources, and curricula in a variety of formats, as well as brief online videos to supplement health topic content. Content is disseminated through its own Web site, local and state health departments, academic institutions, addiction treatment programs, and other partners. E-blasts, online webinars, and social media are additional ways information is disseminated. The site has many offerings for its 3 primary audiences: teens, educators, and parents.

Educators

The Educators page (https://bit.ly/NIDAEducators) provides lessons and activities that elevate evidence-based resources on drugs and addiction that are standards- and skills-driven to help facilitate learning for students served by K–12 educators and counselors, college professors and instructors, and educators/parents/caregivers in homeschool settings. The latest resources include:

- Nurturing my mental health
  - Supports teens in developing healthy coping skills for managing stress and challenging circumstances in the future.
  - Educates teens on how to practice health-enhancing behaviors, such as mindfulness, which can support the management of stress and reduce the chances of exploring substance use as an alternative.
- Is this legit? accessing valid and reliable health information
  - Health literacy can play a role in how teens interpret messages about alcohol and other substances and can shape their expectations about what may happen if they consume drugs and alcohol.
  - Supports teens in developing skills in analyzing, evaluating, and comparing different sources of health information to empower them to reject misinformation and make choices to access evidence-based content.

Parents

The Parents page (https://bit.ly/NIDAParents) provides information and resources, such as Start A Conversation: 10 Questions Teens Ask About Drugs and Health, to help parents to talk with their teens about drugs and their effects and where to go for assistance if needed.

In addition, NIDA for Teens offers resources and activity ideas for those who participate in National Drug and Alcohol Facts Week (NDAFW) (https://bit.ly/NDAFWeek). Launched in 2010, NDAFW is an annual, week-long, health observance that inspires dialogue about the science of drug use and addiction among teens. It provides an opportunity to bring together scientists, students, educators, HCPs, and community partners—to help advance the science and improve the prevention and awareness of substance use in communities and nationwide.

SUMMARY AND FUTURE DIRECTIONS

Timely and wide translation of science and research findings educates providers, informs policy makers and consumers, and ultimately improves public health. Learning from our experiences outlined above, our emphasis for effective dissemination has been to build and leverage partnerships among various stakeholders; to seek and apply the input of our partners and audiences to inform content development and dissemination; and to make content readily accessible, user-friendly, clearly articulated and reproducible with no fees levied. Building on our current partnerships we plan to enhance dissemination and explore a few new directions:

- Partnering with national organizations representing diversity in medicine and other health professional disciplines could help increase the visibility and importance of serving these populations

- Enhancing our outreach to child psychiatrists, adolescent medicine providers, nurse practitioners, and physician assistants, and expanding the target audiences to include pediatricians, dentists, and pharmacists.
- Expanding communication efforts beyond the primary care community to include tailored messaging to providers in other settings whereby youth receive care, such as emergency departments, school-based health care, and homeless health care.
- Performing due diligence to provide the most relevant, useful, and timely information to providers to fill gaps in current knowledge. Through formative research with researchers, our partners in professional organization and HCP panels, we will continue to seek input and feedback to further improve our dissemination efforts

We hope this sets the stage for a call to HCPs to educate youth on the dangers of substance use, and to treat youth who may have already developed a SUD.

DISCLAIMER

This article reflects the views of the authors and may not reflect the opinions, views, and official policy or position of the US Department of Health and Human Services or any of its affiliated institutions or agencies.

ACKNOWLEDGMENTS

This work was supported in part by the National Institute on Drug Abuse, United States under contract number 75N95020C00028RFP (CTN Dissemination Initiative, the Bizzell Group, LLC); 75N95020C00006 (Outreach and Education to Health Care Providers on Substance use, JBS International). The authors thank David Liu, Erika Capinguian, and Ashley Matus for their contributions.

DISCLOSURE

Drs G.A. Subramaniam and K. Huntley, Mss Q. Blackeney, M. Corbin, and J. Linton are employees of the National Institute on Drug Abuse. Dr G.A. Subramaniam, Mss M. Corbin, J. Linton, and Q. Blackeney have no other conflicts to report. Dr K. Huntley's spouse is eligible for a defined benefit plan through Pfizer from previous employment. L. Nolan is an employee of JBS International and has no conflicts to report. Dr T. Mandell and Ms K. Crenshaw are employees of the Bizzell Group and have no conflicts to report.

REFERENCES

1. Morris ZS, Wooding S, Grant J. The answer is 17 years, what is the question: understanding time lags in translational research. J R Soc Med 2011;104(12): 510–20. Accessed December 14, 2021.

2. NIH policy on the dissemination of NIH-funded clinical trial information. Available at: https://grants.nih.gov/policy/clinical-trials/reporting/understanding/nih-policy. htm. Accessed December 14, 2021.

3. Levy S, Weiss R, Sherritt L, et al. An electronic screen for triaging adolescent substance use by risk levels. JAMA Pediatr 2014;168(9):822–8. Accessed December 14, 2021.

4. Kelly SM, Gryczynski J, Mitchell SG, et al. Validity of brief screening instrument for adolescent tobacco, alcohol, and drug use. Pediatrics 2014;133(5):819–26. Accessed December 14, 2021.

5. Lanken PN, Novack DH, Daetwyler C, et al. Efficacy of an internet-based learning module and small-group debriefing on trainees' attitudes and communication skills toward patients with substance use disorders: results of a cluster randomized controlled trial. Acad Med 2015;90(3):345–54. Accessed December 14, 2021.

6. Yang LH, Wong LY, Grivel MM, et al. Stigma and substance use disorders: an international phenomenon. Curr Opin Psychiatry 2017;30(5):378–88. Accessed December 14, 2021.

7. Ashford RD, Brown AM, McDaniel J, et al. Biased labels: an experimental study of language and stigma among individuals in recovery and health professionals. Subst Use Misuse 2019;54(8):1376–84. Accessed December 14, 2021.

8. Carney T, Myers B. Effectiveness of early interventions for substance-using adolescents: findings from a systematic review and meta-analysis. Subst Abuse Treat Prev Policy 2012;7:25–39. December 15, 2021.

9. Johnston LD, Miech RA, O'Malley PM, et al. Monitoring the Future national survey results on drug use 1975-2020: overview, key findings on adolescent drug use. Ann Arbor: institute for Social Research, University of Michigan. Available at: https://files.eric.ed.gov/fulltext/ED611736.pdf. Accessed December 14, 2021.

10. Twenge JM, Cooper AB, Joiner TE, et al. Age, period, and cohort trends in mood disorder indicators and suicide-related outcomes in a nationally representative dataset, 2005-2017. J Abnorm Psychol 2019;128(3):185–99. Accessed December 14, 2021.

11. Miron O, Yu K, Wilf-Miron R, et al. Suicide rates among adolescents and young adults in the United States, 2000-2017. JAMA 2019;321(23):2362–4. Accessed December 14, 2021.

Epilogue

Paula Riggs, MD

We wish to thank the authors for their important contributions to this issue. The main goal of this issue is to provide clinician readers with clinically meaningful research-based information about adolescent cannabis use and psychoeducation resources for youth and families (Geetha A. Subramaniam and colleagues' article, "National Institute on Drug Abuse: Dissemination of Scientific Knowledge to Improve Adolescent Health," in this issue). It is especially important for behavioral health clinicians and pediatric primary care providers to have a sound science-based understanding of the adverse effects of adolescent cannabis use on neurocognitive development (J. Cobb Scott's article, "Impact of Adolescent Cannabis Use on Neurocognitive and Brain Development," in this issue), mental health problems (Karla Molinero and Jesse D. Hinckley's article, "Adolescent Cannabis Use, Comorbid ADHD, and Other Internalizing and Externalizing Disorders," in this issue), and dose-dependent impact on poorer psychosocial and functional outcomes (Jonathan D. Schaefer and colleagues', "The Effects of Adolescent Cannabis Use on Psychosocial Functioning: A Critical Review of the Evidence," in this issue).[1] Although it is still too early to determine the full public health impact of cannabis legalization, thus far legalization has not been associated with a significant increase in the overall prevalence of adolescent cannabis use. However, cannabis legalization is associated with a decrease in adolescents' perception of harm associated with regular cannabis use (Kristie Ladegard and Devika Bhatia' s article, "Impact of Cannabis Legalization on Adolescent Cannabis Use," in this issue). There is also little doubt that cannabis legalization and commercialization have increased the availability and access to extremely-high-potency cannabis products in both adolescents and adults (Kristie Ladegard and Devika Bhatia' s article, "Impact of Cannabis Legalization on Adolescent Cannabis Use," in this issue). As the market share of high-potency cannabis products continues to grow, so has their use among adolescents. Increased use of high-potency cannabis concentrates among adolescents is thought to be a significant contributor to increasing rates of cannabis-related problems and cannabis use disorder in young people. States that have legalized cannabis have consistently reported increases in the number of cannabis-related emergency room visits (eg, psychosis, hyperemesis), hospitalizations, suicidality, and motor vehicle accidents in adolescents and adults (Kristie Ladegard and Devika Bhatia' s article, "Impact of Cannabis Legalization on Adolescent Cannabis Use"; and Daniel Hashemi and Kevin Gray's article, "Cannabis Use Disorder in Adolescents"; and Jonathan D. Schaefer and colleagues', "The Effects of Adolescent Cannabis Use on Psychosocial Functioning: A Critical

This article originally appeared in *Child and Adolescent Psychiatric Clinics*, Volume 32 Issue 1, January 2023.
Division of Addiction Science, Prevention, and Treatment, Department of Psychiatry, University of Colorado School of Medicine, 3434 Jennings Street, San Diego, CA 92106, USA
E-mail address: paula.riggs@cuanschutz.edu

Review of the Evidence"; and Karla Molinero and Jesse D. Hinckley's article, "Adolescent Cannabis Use, Comorbid ADHD, and Other Internalizing and Externalizing Disorders"; and Michelle L. West and Shadi Sharif's article, "Cannabis and Psychosis"; and Abigail L. Tuvel and colleagues' article, "A Review of the Effects of Adolescent Cannabis Use on Physical Health," in this issue.)

On December 7, 2021, the US Surgeon General, Vivek Murthy, issued a national advisory identifying the urgent need to address the nation's youth mental health crisis. Pediatric health experts have called the current youth mental health crisis a national emergency. However, the contribution of adolescent cannabis use to this crisis is often understated and underappreciated. Jonathan D. Schaefer and colleagues', "The Effects of Adolescent Cannabis Use on Psychosocial Functioning: A Critical Review of the Evidence"; and Karla Molinero and Jesse D. Hinckley's article, "Adolescent Cannabis Use, Comorbid ADHD, and Other Internalizing and Externalizing Disorders," in this issue address the strong relationship between adolescent cannabis use and mental health problems, including increased risk of psychosis, depression, anxiety disorders, as well as suicidal thoughts and behaviors. Cannabis use before age 17 years significantly increases the risk of progression to cannabis use disorder as well as the risk of becoming addicted to other substances tried later, including methamphetamine, other illicit substances, and opioids (Daniel Hashemi and Kevin Gray's article, "Cannabis Use Disorder in Adolescents," in this issue).[2] In the current climate, these substances are increasingly likely to be contaminated with fentanyl, often with deadly consequences. There is also great concern about the increasing number of recent reports of unintentional overdose deaths in adolescents due to fentanyl-contaminated cannabis. Rates of unintentional overdose deaths (mostly fentanyl) in young people have increased dramatically in the past 5 years.[3] A recent study reported more than 1.5 million years of life lost from unintentional opioid overdose, mostly due to fentanyl, among 12- to 24-year-olds between 2015 and 2019.[3,4]

These concerning trends, in the context of the ongoing opioid crisis, expanding legalized cannabis environment, and the current youth mental health crisis, underscore the critical importance of early identification and prevention to reduce risk factors for adolescent cannabis use and associated mental health problems. Paula D. Riggs's article, "A Pragmatic Clinical Approach to Substance Abuse Prevention," in this issue on prevention provides clinicians with the "common elements" of evidence-based prevention interventions in an effort to encourage their utilization and application beyond school-based settings. These common prevention elements address risk factors that arise in early childhood and that have been identified as common antecedent risk factors for mental health problems and substance misuse by adolescence. Addressing the current youth mental health crisis will also require more robust efforts to expand access and the availability of evidence-based mental health and substance prevention and treatment (Zachary W. Adams and colleagues' article, "Treatment of Adolescent Cannabis Use Disorders," in this issue). Now, more than ever, there is an urgent need to redouble efforts to break down silos between substance and mental health treatment. This will require further development of more workable and efficient coordinated care models, with the longer-term goal of fully integrating mental health and substance treatment within the health care system. Meaningful progress toward achieving this goal will require significant additional resources and a sustained commitment to address the critical shortage of clinicians with mental health and addiction training. It is important to note that progress will likely continue to be painstakingly slow and incremental without significant behavioral health payment reforms.

Addressing the current youth mental health crisis, underpinned by the ever-expanding environment of legalized cannabis and the ongoing opioid crisis, the effects of which are increasingly impacting adolescents, will require an "all hands on deck" approach. The overarching goal of this issue is to provide clinicians working in schools, pediatric primary care, and behavioral health settings with research-based information and practical clinical skills and tools that can be applied in a broad range of clinical settings to improve substance screening, prevention, and early intervention. Unfortunately, this alone will not be enough. Clinicians, programs, and agencies must develop innovative approaches to overcome addiction-related stigma and the entrenched systemic and economic forces that sustain existing treatment silos. Jessica B Calihan and Sharon Levy's article, "Substance Use Screening, Brief Intervention, and Referral to Treatment in Pediatric Primary Care, School-based Health Clinics & Mental Health Clinics"; and Ken C. Winters and colleagues' article, "Brief Interventions for Cannabis Using Adolescents," in this issue highlight the substantial progress and widespread adoption of screening, brief intervention, and referral to treatment (SBIRT) protocols that have expanded substance screening and implementation of brief motivationally enhancing interventions for adolescent substance misuse in school-based and pediatric primary care settings. Zachary W. Adams and colleagues' article, "Treatment of Adolescent Cannabis Use Disorders," in this issue identifies the growing number of evidence-based adolescent substance treatment interventions with proven efficacy. Unfortunately, there has been limited progress in our collective efforts to expand access and the availability of these high-quality evidence-based substance treatment interventions and almost no progress toward increasing adolescent substance treatment engagement and utilization in the past decade. Still, fewer than 10% of adolescents who could benefit from substance treatment receive it. The majority of those who do are in community-based substance treatment programs that largely serve youth referred by social services or the juvenile justice system. Yet, the vast majority (>90%) of adolescents with a substance use disorders are still in school and/or have a pediatric primary care provider and most are not (yet) involved with juvenile justice. Engaging such youth (ie, non-court-mandated) in substance treatment will require the development of more innovative "warm handoff" treatment referral approaches. In clinical settings that do not have integrated or colocated adolescent substance treatment services, it is important to develop a meaningful partnership with one or more substance treatment programs or providers followed by collaborative development of "warm handoff" referral procedures for adolescents who screen positive for problematic substance use or substance use disorders. It is important to keep in mind that adolescents who screen positive for problematic cannabis/substance use disorders are not likely to jump at the chance to enroll in substance treatment when referred. Existing adolescent substance treatment referral procedures based on substance screening, even using standardized SBIRT protocols, generally result in low rates of substance treatment engagement among referred youth. In an effort to overcome barriers to adolescent substance treatment engagement, we are currently piloting a promising alternative using a motivationally enhancing direct outreach approach. Instead of referring adolescents who screen positive for monthly, weekly, or more frequent cannabis/substance use to treatment, we ask our pediatric and school-based referral partners to express concern about the frequency of substance use based on screening results and ask the adolescent if it would be ok to share their substance screening results with an expert, who would call the teen for a brief (10- to 15-minute) confidential telephone evaluation/consultation. Most adolescents agree to a brief confidential telephone consultation, in which the "expert" consultant uses an empathic motivational interviewing approach to explore the adolescent's ambivalence regarding behavior change and to provide psychoeducation information about ENCOMPASS—our integrated mental health/substance treatment program (motivational enhancement therapy/cognitive behavioral therapy [MET/CBT] + contingency management [CM]). Thus far, using this direct outreach approach known as SBIRE (ie, screening, brief intervention, and referral for brief evaluation), on average 40% of referred youth are engaging in substance treatment, defined as showing up for at least 1 substance treatment appointment (Riggs, unpublished data, 2022). These preliminary data are sufficiently promising to warrant further exploration and research. The SBIRE approach is described in a Charting Pediatrics podcast interview: "When Substance Use Disorders Come to Pediatrics" (S4:E16) and also presented at a Clinical Perspectives Symposium, "You've Screened, Now What?" at the 68th American Academy of Child and Adolescent Psychiatry (AACAP) Annual Meeting in 2021.

We strongly encourage other clinicians to collaboratively develop and pilot similar innovative warm handoff referral procedures, adapted for your clinical settings, to facilitate adolescent substance treatment engagement. We also hope that clinicians will find the research-based information in this issue to be clinically useful and use the practical skills and resources provided to improve the prevention, early intervention, and treatment of adolescents with cannabis use disorders in your clinical practice settings. We also hope that this issue will inspire the development of new and innovative coordinated and integrated care models that will spur us toward a more fully integrated health care system, accessible to all.

FUNDING

Dr. Riggs is Co-PI (Principal Investigator) on a current NIDA grant 1 R01 DA053288-01: "Evaluation of Clinical Effectiveness, Cost, and Implementation Factors to Optimize Scalability of Treatment for Co-occurring SUD and PTSD Among Teens". 2021-2026 National Institute on Drug Abuse (NIDA) R01NIDA.

REFERENCES

1. Copeland WE, Hill SW, Shanahan L. Adult psychiatric, substance, and functional outcomes of different definitions of early cannabis use. J Am Acad Child Adolesc Psychiatry 2022;61(4):533–43.
2. Olfson M, Wall MM, Liu S, et al. Cannabis use and risk of prescription opioid use disorder in the United States. Am J Psychiatry 2018;175(1):47–53.
3. Hall TO, Trimble C, Garcia S, et al. Unintentional drug overdose mortality in years of life lost among adolescents and young people in the US from 2015-2019. Research Letter. JAMA Pediatr 2022;176(4):415–7.
4. Charting pediatrics: when substance use disorder comes to pediatrics with Debbie Singer M.D. and Paula Riggs M.D. E4; S16, January 12, 2021. https://chartingpediatrics.libsyn.com/when-substance-abuse-disorders-come-to-pediatrics-with-debbie-singer-md-paula-riggs-md-s4e16.

UNITED STATES POSTAL SERVICE®

Statement of Ownership, Management, and Circulation (All Periodicals Publications Except Requester Publications)

1. Publication Title	2. Publication Number	3. Filing Date
PSYCHIATRIC CLINICS OF NORTH AMERICA	000 – 703	9/18/2023

4. Issue Frequency	5. Number of Issues Published Annually	6. Annual Subscription Price
MAR, JUN, SEP, DEC	4	$352.00

7. Complete Mailing Address of Known Office of Publication (Not printer) (Street, city, county, state, and ZIP+4®)

ELSEVIER INC.
230 Park Avenue, Suite 800
New York, NY 10169

Contact Person
Malathi Samayan

Telephone (Include area code)
91-44-4299-4507

8. Complete Mailing Address of Headquarters or General Business Office of Publisher (Not printer)

ELSEVIER INC.
230 Park Avenue, Suite 800
New York, NY 10169

9. Full Names and Complete Mailing Addresses of Publisher, Editor, and Managing Editor (Do not leave blank)

Publisher (Name and complete mailing address)
DOLORES MELONI, ELSEVIER INC.
1600 JOHN F KENNEDY BLVD. SUITE 1600
PHILADELPHIA, PA 19103-2899

Editor (Name and complete mailing address)
MEGAN ASHDOWN, ELSEVIER INC.
1600 JOHN F KENNEDY BLVD. SUITE 1600
PHILADELPHIA, PA 19103-2899

Managing Editor (Name and complete mailing address)
PATRICK MANLEY, ELSEVIER INC.
1600 JOHN F KENNEDY BLVD. SUITE 1600
PHILADELPHIA, PA 19103-2899

10. Owner (Do not leave blank. If the publication is owned by a corporation, give the name and address of the corporation immediately followed by the names and addresses of all stockholders owning or holding 1 percent or more of the total amount of stock. If not owned by a corporation, give the names and addresses of the individual owners. If owned by a partnership or other unincorporated firm, give its name and address as well as those of each individual owner. If the publication is published by a nonprofit organization, give its name and address.)

Full Name	Complete Mailing Address
WHOLLY OWNED SUBSIDIARY OF REED/ELSEVIER, US HOLDINGS	1600 JOHN F KENNEDY BLVD. SUITE 1600 PHILADELPHIA, PA 19103-2899

11. Known Bondholders, Mortgagees, and Other Security Holders Owning or Holding 1 Percent or More of Total Amount of Bonds, Mortgages, or Other Securities. If none, check box. → ☐ None

Full Name	Complete Mailing Address
N/A	

12. Tax Status (For completion by nonprofit organizations authorized to mail at nonprofit rates.) (Check one)
The purpose, function, and nonprofit status of this organization and the exempt status for federal income tax purposes:
☒ Has Not Changed During Preceding 12 Months
☐ Has Changed During Preceding 12 Months (Publisher must submit explanation of change with this statement)

PS Form 3526, July 2014 [Page 1 of 4 (see instructions page 4)] PSN: 7530-01-000-9931 PRIVACY NOTICE: See our privacy policy on www.usps.com.

---

13. Publication Title		14. Issue Date for Circulation Data Below
PSYCHIATRIC CLINICS OF NORTH AMERICA		JUNE 2023

15. Extent and Nature of Circulation			Average No. Copies Each Issue During Preceding 12 Months	No. Copies of Single Issue Published Nearest to Filing Date
a. Total Number of Copies (Net press run)			128	122
b. Paid Circulation (By Mail and Outside the Mail)	(1)	Mailed Outside-County Paid Subscriptions Stated on PS Form 3541 (Include paid distribution above nominal rate, advertiser's proof copies, and exchange copies)	71	76
	(2)	Mailed In-County Paid Subscriptions Stated on PS Form 3541 (Include paid distribution above nominal rate, advertiser's proof copies, and exchange copies)	0	0
	(3)	Paid Distribution Outside the Mails Including Sales Through Dealers and Carriers, Street Vendors, Counter Sales, and Other Paid Distribution Outside USPS®	41	3
	(4)	Paid Distribution by Other Classes of Mail Through the USPS (e.g., First-Class Mail®)	15	12
c. Total Paid Distribution (Sum of 15b (1), (2), (3), and (4))		▶	127	121
d. Free or Nominal Rate Distribution (By Mail and Outside the Mail)	(1)	Free or Nominal Rate Outside-County Copies included on PS Form 3541	1	1
	(2)	Free or Nominal Rate In-County Copies Included on PS Form 3541	0	0
	(3)	Free or Nominal Rate Copies Mailed at Other Classes Through the USPS (e.g., First-Class Mail)	0	0
	(4)	Free or Nominal Rate Distribution Outside the Mail (Carriers or other means)	0	0
e. Total Free or Nominal Rate Distribution (Sum of 15d (1), (2), (3) and (4))		▶	1	1
f. Total Distribution (Sum of 15c and 15e)		▶	128	122
g. Copies not Distributed (See Instructions to Publishers #4 (page #3))		▶	0	0
h. Total (Sum of 15f and g)		▶	128	122
i. Percent Paid (15c divided by 15f times 100)		▶	99.22%	99.18%

* If you are claiming electronic copies, go to line 16 on page 3. If you are not claiming electronic copies, skip to line 17 on page 3.

PS Form 3526, July 2014 (Page 2 of 4)

16. Electronic Copy Circulation		Average No. Copies Each Issue During Preceding 12 Months	No. Copies of Single Issue Published Nearest to Filing Date
a. Paid Electronic Copies	▶		
b. Total Paid Print Copies (Line 15c) + Paid Electronic Copies (Line 16a)	▶		
c. Total Print Distribution (Line 15f) + Paid Electronic Copies (Line 16a)	▶		
d. Percent Paid (Both Print & Electronic Copies) (16b divided by 16c × 100)	▶		

☒ I certify that 50% of all my distributed copies (electronic and print) are paid above a nominal price.

17. Publication of Statement of Ownership

☒ If the publication is a general publication, publication of this statement is required. Will be printed ☐ Publication not required.

in the DECEMBER 2023 issue of this publication.

18. Signature and Title of Editor, Publisher, Business Manager, or Owner	Date
Malathi Samayan Malathi Samayan - Distribution Controller	9/18/2023

I certify that all information furnished on this form is true and complete. I understand that anyone who furnishes false or misleading information on this form or who omits material or information requested on the form may be subject to criminal sanctions (including fines and imprisonment) and/or civil sanctions (including civil penalties).

PS Form 3526, July 2014 (Page 3 of 4) PRIVACY NOTICE: See our privacy policy on www.usps.com

Moving?

Make sure your subscription moves with you!

To notify us of your new address, find your **Clinics Account Number** (located on your mailing label above your name), and contact customer service at:

Email: journalscustomerservice-usa@elsevier.com

800-654-2452 (subscribers in the U.S. & Canada)
314-447-8871 (subscribers outside of the U.S. & Canada)

Fax number: 314-447-8029

Elsevier Health Sciences Division
Subscription Customer Service
3251 Riverport Lane
Maryland Heights, MO 63043

*To ensure uninterrupted delivery of your subscription, please notify us at least 4 weeks in advance of move.

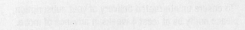

Printed and bound by CPI Group (UK) Ltd, Croydon, CR0 4YY

03/10/2024

01040469-0017